Sport Medicine: Protection, Treatment and Nutrition

A Volume in MSS' Series on Sport Medicine

Papers by
Russell M. Lane, Leonard A. Larson, Anderson
Spickard et al.

MSS Information Corporation
655 Madison Avenue, New York, N.Y. 10021

Library of Congress Cataloging in Publication Data

Main entry under title:

Sport medicine.

    1. Sports medicine--Addresses, essays, lectures.
I. Lane, Russell M. [DNLM: 1. Athletic injuries--
Prevention & control--Coll. wks. 3. Sport medicine--
Collected works. QT260 L266s 1973]
RC1215.S65   617'.1027   73-10420
ISBN 0-8422-7140-6

TABLE OF CONTENTS

CREDITS AND ACKNOWLEDGEMENTS

Abraham, Joseph N., "Trainer's Role in High School Athletics," *New York State Journal of Medicine*, 1970, 70:537-542.

Gillen, H. William, "Needs for Diving Accident Information," *Archives of Environmental Health*, 1967, 14:517.

Harwood, Mark R.; and Gerald L. Strange, "Orthopedic Aspects and Safety Factors in Snow Skiing," *New York State Journal of Medicine*, 1966, 66:2899-2907.

Henderson, Edward D.; and Donald J. Erickson, "Preseason Conditioning Exercises for High School Football Players," *Minnesota Medicine*, 1967, 50:1263-1271.

Lane, Russell M., "Uniform Code of Medical Qualifications for Participation in Interscholastic Athletics in Maine," *Journal of the Maine Medical Association*, 1969, 60:247-254 passim.

Larson, Leonard A., "An International Research Program for the Standardization of Physical Fitness Tests," *Journal of Sport Medicine*, 1966, 6:259-261.

Lindbergh, Jon, "The Need for Practical Methods of Presymptomatic Bubble Detection," *Journal of Occupational Medicine*, 1969, 11:278-280.

Maganzini, Herman C., "Weight Control in Athletics," *Maryland State Medical Journal*, 1969, 18:77-80.

Manfredi, Daniel H., "Sports Medicine in Urban New York," *New York State Journal of Medicine*, 1967, 67:2381-2384.

Ryan, Allan J., "The Physician in the Training Room," *Archives of Physical Medicine*, 1968, 49:340-342.

Savastano, A.A., "The Team Physician and the Law," *Rhode Island Medical Journal*, 1968, 51:558-560 passim.

Spickard, Anderson, "Heat Stroke in College Football and Suggestions for Prevention," *Southern Medical Journal*, 1968, 61:791-796.

Spickard, Anderson; and Joe Worden, "How to Prevent Heat Stroke in Football Players," *Southern Medical Journal*, 1968, 61:897-903.

Stiles, Merritt H., "Injury Prevention in Skiing and Snowmobiling," *Northwest Medicine*, 1972, 71:29-32.

Stiles, Merritt H., "Medical Preparation for the Olympic Games," *Journal of the American Medical Association*, 1968, 205:771-774.

Suker, Jacob R., "The Medical Aspects of Professional Baseball," *Illinois Medical Journal*, 1970, 137:89-92.

Tucker, Richard; and Gordon C. Lipe, "Safety in a Release Binding," *Industrial Medicine and Surgery*, 1967, 36:30-34.

Turco, S.J.P., "Diets in Athletics," *Rhode Island Medical Journal*, 1969, 52:325-326.

Williams, J.G.P., "Nutrition in Sport," *The Practitioner*, 1968, 201: 324-329.

PREFACE

This volume, part of MSS' Series on Sport Medicine, contains studies on the control and prevention of athletic injuries. Due to the current emphasis on physical fitness and the rapid growth of amateur and professional participation in a variety of sports, many physicians are devoting full time to medical supervision and care of athletes.

Measures for avoiding heat stroke in football players, conditioning exercises for school athletes, medical preparation for olympic games, and safety factors in snow-mobiling, skiing, and diving are the topics discussed in this volume. The role of the team physician and trainer in scholastic and professional sports, and nutritional factors in treating the athlete are also examined.

Protective Equipment and Other Preventive Measures

Uniform Code of Medical Qualifications for Participants in Interscholastic Athletics in Maine

RUSSELL M. LANE, M.D.

The United States has traditionally been a sports-oriented nation and since World War II, we, as a people, have increasingly given recognition to the importance of sports and physical fitness in the character development and health maintenance of our population. Since organized athletics on the secondary school level ("Interscholastics") encompasses the greatest numerical and most accessible group of our youth in probably their most sensitive years for both physical growth and character development, we naturally turn our attention towards medical guidelines for said interscholastic sports participation. These medical guidelines are herewith formulated into this CODE, whose purpose is to give direction to state and community leaders, who are in positions to translate guidelines to actual practices, which will in turn directly effect the health and safety of our youth in their athletic pursuits. In so formulating this CODE, we all must fully realize that although sports have real health and education values, said values are not assumed without some forms of supervision and control. In the formulation, our primary commitment has been the same expressed by Dr. Thomas Quigley of Harvard in 1957; namely, that each sports participant is entitled to good medical care and good health supervision as part of his (or her) involvement in an organized athletic program.

ITEM I – THE RECORD FORMS FOR MEDICAL HISTORY
AND PHYSICAL EXAMINATION, THE STUDENT-
PARTICIPATION AND PARENTAL-CONSENT FORM

The accompanying forms (Appendices A, B and C) are self-explanatory regarding the requested information. Their format and content represent the combined thinking of the American Medical Association's Committee on the Medical Aspects of Sports and of the National Federation of State High School Athletic Associations, with some minor adjustments for most suitable use in Maine. It is essential that all interscholastic athletic candidates have all three forms completed and submitted to their school office annually, and that said annual evaluation be done prior to the first practice of the earliest sport in the academic year for which the student is a candidate. The completed forms are to be maintained in the school office during the student's stay in high school and for four years thereafter: – the 'Participation and Consent' form, for school administrative review, and the medical forms for appropriate review and use as medical records by the school physician or nurse, and by the athletic team-physician if there be one per se. The advantages of uncomplicated, standardized, medically-competent forms for all schools and all sports should be obvious to everyone concerned. Whether the medical history and examination is done by the student's family doctor or done by the school or team doctor, and whether the expenses involved are borne by the student and his (or her) parents or by the school; these matters are strictly not within the jurisdiction of this CODE, and must be decided within each individual school system for itself.

ITEM II – GROUPING OF SPORTS BY COMPETITIVE
CHARACTERISTICS

Although recognizing that all sports have their individual characteristics and their unique physical and mental demands on their participants, it is rather universally acknowledged that we have three general categories of

11

competitive athletics. These broad groupings will be most helpful in establishing the workability of this CODE: and are listed with those organized interscholastic sports of Maine in each category:

Contact Sports	Endurance Sports (non-contact)	Leisure Sports
football	cross country	golf
basketball	skiing	bowling
baseball	swimming	archery
soccer	track and field	riflery
wrestling	tennis	sailing
lacrosse	volleyball	
ice hockey	gymnastics	
softball (girls)	crew	
field hockey (girls)	fencing	

It is imperative to note that the benefits of sports toward fitness, health, and character are as applicable to *girls* as they are to boys, and that this CODE is intended to apply equally to both sexes. Hopefully, we will see increasingly more programs in interscholastic athletics for our female youth, with resultant increasing beneficial effects in the factors mentioned above.

ITEM III – GENERAL DISCUSSION OF QUALIFYING
VERSUS DISQUALIFYING MEDICAL CONDITIONS
AND CIRCUMSTANCES

The commitments of the physician in this area of athletic medicine are twofold: 1) to withhold the athlete from participation if medical reasons for such action are present, and 2) to prevent unwarranted medical disqualification of any athlete with the desire for participation. Said physician in athletic medicine must never lose sight of this second commitment; he must have the courage to make decisions in this sphere, without shielding his ignorance and indecision in ultra-conservative disqualification or inaction.

Under the heading of the physician's first commitment above, the major reasons for restricting participation will be: a) when there is a disease or process which would prevent the athlete from participating and competing fairly with 'normal' persons; and b) when there is a disease or process which might be significantly and/or permanently aggravated by participation. Let it be further urged that potential athletes with obvious deficiences which preclude contact or endurance sports, be identified

APPENDIX A

MEDICAL HISTORY QUESTIONNAIRE FOR SPORTS CANDIDATES
(to be completed by parents)

Name: Date of birth:

Home address:

Parents' name: Telephone number:

1. Significant past injuries (fractures, dislocations, concussions, major lacerations)

2. Major medical illnesses (tuberculosis, rheumatic fever, asthma, diabetes, epilepsy, jaundice, etc.)

3. Currently taking medication?   What?

    Currently under a doctor's care?   For what?

4. Wear glasses?   or Contact Lenses?

5. Wear removable dentures (or bridgework)?   or dental braces?

6. Any significant allergies? (foods, stinging insects, drugs, hives, asthma, other)

7. Any previous surgery?   or medical hospitalizations?

8. Tetanus toxoid, initial series   (Yes or No)

    Tetanus toxoid, most recent booster – date (   )

9. Oral (Sabin) Polio Vaccine, initial series (Yes or No)

    Oral (Sabin) Polio Vaccine, Tri-Valent booster (Yes or No)

10. Do you know of any reason why this student should not participate in interscholastic athletics?   Explain.

Date: ....

                                           (Parent's or Guardian's signature)

13

MEDICAL EXAMINATION
(to be completed by examining physician)

Name of student
Grade   Age
General appearance
Head
Eyes: general
Ears: general
Respiratory
Cardiovascular
Liver   Spleen
Musculoskeletal
Neurological
Genitalia
Laboratory: Urinalysis
               Other, if indicated
Immunizations: Tetanus Toxoid

Height   Weight   School   Blood Pressure
                                Pulse

                Nose & Throat
                Vision: R 20/   ; L 20/
                Hearing: R -   ; L -

                                        Hernia
                Skin
                Psychiatric

                Oral Tri-Val. Polio

Comments:

"I certify that I have on this date examined this student and that, on the basis of the examination requested by the school authorities and the student's medical history as furnished to me, I have found no reason which would make it medically inadvisable for this student to compete in supervised athletic activities, EXCEPT THOSE CROSSED OUT BELOW."

Contact Sports: football, basketball, baseball, soccer, wrestling, ice hockey, lacrosse, girls' softball, girls' field hockey.

Endurance Sports: cross country, skiing, swimming, track & field, tennis, volleyball, gymnastics, crew.

Leisure Sports: golf, bowling, archery, riflery, sailing.

Estimated desirable weight level for wrestling: .... pounds.

Signed: ....
                                    (examining physician)

Printed name: ....

Telephone: ....

Date of Exam: ....

14

as early as possible in their school careers and directed towards less vigorous sports, for which they can qualify. Chronologically early re-direction will usually result in a devoted athlete at his (or her) new and medically appropriate level in the sports spectrum, and will be a rewarding experience for all involved.

In performing the medical evaluation, the physician must exercise thoughtful judgment to arrive at his decision for or against athletic participation by the candidate. The decision must include accurate diagnoses, a reasonable knowledge of any encountered pathological process, a thorough background of information of the many types of sports and the psycho-physiological demands of each, and a full evaluation of the personality of the candidate. The decision which includes these factors will be a wise one; but omitting any of them could prove harmful to the athlete, to the team, to the physicians, and to sports in general.

A. *"Matching"* – This term refers to the usually desirable practice of grouping participants on the basis of comparable levels of physical size and emotional maturation. The factors of size and maturity are often hard to delineate, since they involve individual judgment to so great an extent. They will be less problematical as more and more schools develop the sorely needed interscholastic junior varsity and freshman sports programs, thereby providing athletic participation for an increasing number and spectrum of students.

In the specific area of the varsity football squad, the minimum candidate weight is suggested to be 125 lbs. at the pre-season medical evaluation, and the minimum squad size for each interscholastic contest is suggested to be at least 22, "dressed and able," regular team members.

Furthermore, in the specific area of wrestling, the practice of an athlete competing markedly above his "desirable weight level" (see Appendix B) or of sweating and starving himself down for a match markedly below said level, is to be vigorously condemned as potentially medically harmful and contrary to the true intent of all sports participation. Consequently, a sincere effort is urged upon all physicians completing Appendix B for a potential interscholastic wrestler, to arrive at the "desirable weight level" for the student in question with full consideration of the fact that it will represent their considered medical appraisal of what the weight would ideally be when the student is in good condition for athletic competition, namely wrestling. It would then be considered reasonable to restrict each wrestler to competition

APPENDIX C

STUDENT PARTICIPATION & PARENTAL APPROVAL FORM

Full name of student:

Name of school:

Date signed:

Date of birth:

Place of birth:

This application to compete in interscholastic athletics for the above-named high school is entirely voluntary on my part and is made with the understanding that I have not violated any of the eligibility rules and regulations of the Maine State Principals' Association.

Student's Signature: ....

"I hereby give my consent for the above-named student: (1) to represent his school in athletic activities, except those crossed out on the accompanying form by the examining physician, provided that such athletic activities are approved by the Maine State Principals' Association; (2) to accompany any school team of which he is a member on any of its local or out-of-town trips. I authorize the school to obtain, through a physician of its own choice, any emergency medical care that may become reasonably necessary for the student in the course of such athletic activities or such travel. I also agree not to hold the school or anyone acting in its behalf responsible for any injury occurring to the above-named student in the course of such athletic activities or such travel."

Date signed:

Signature: ....

                   (Parent or Guardian)

Address: .... (Street)

                                   (City/Town)

Note: 1) These associated forms (3) must be filled out completely and filed in the school principal's office before the student will be allowed to draw equipment, to practice, or to compete in interscholastic athletics. In addition to these three (3) standard forms, any individual school may have other specific requirements of their prospective athletes.

2) All interscholastic athletic participants are required to have an in-force, accident-coverage, insurance program approved by their school prior to the onset of their sports season and continuing therethrough.

16

in the class closest to his listed "desirable weight level," and to allow him to compete one class above or move one class below, but no greater deviation from his base during any given season.

B. *Acute Infections* – That the acute phase of an infectious disease (contagious, or not) is a time for restriction from sports participation, will lead to almost no controversy; yet the appropriate period of convalescent restriction will be less easy to decide, and must remain an individual decision by the responsible physician in each situation. Some more common examples of temporarily disqualifying acute infections are: Chickenpox, Mumps, Measles (both kinds), Scarlet fever (or Scarlatina), Rheumatic fever, Respiratory infections, Genitourinary infections, Hepatitis, Infectious mononucleosis, Boils, Furunculosis, Impetigo, Cellulitis, Lymphangitis, Pediculosis, and "Herpes simplex gladiatorum."

C. *Blood and Related Conditions* – The pre-season exam will sometimes uncover these problems and point the way to appropriate treatment; in other cases, the therapy will be well established. Once again, exacting rules for disqualification, or not, will require mature and compassionate medical understanding and judgment, with consideration of all factors involved. (See Item IV C. for recommended specific disease restrictions.)

D. *Diabetes Mellitus* – The tendency for marginal control at best in juvenile diabetics, the increasing desire for sports participation in a growing proportion of our youth (including said juvenile diabetics), and the requirement for having and maintaining adequate control of one's diabetes (if present) prior to being medically qualified for interscholastic sports; these factors should all be appropriately and vigorously 'used' to promote better health in this group of young people.

E. *Eyes* – Vertebrate animals, namely Man in our discussion, are fortunate that their means of vision comes through a *pair* of eyes; for eyes are relatively vulnerable to injury by virtue of their essential nature to almost all activities (thereby being in the center of the action), they are rather hard to devise protective equipment for without impairing their efficiency as organs of sight, and blindness in an eye from injury to said eye is not too unusual, despite good medical treatment. However, we are further fortunate in that eye injuries in sports are usually unilateral (as compared with the bilateral nature usually associated with fire and explosion), and in that a person is able to adjust to a healthy, productive life with only one functioning eye ('monocular vision'). In contrast, total blindness is a most severe handicap, and the direction of reasoning of this CODE will be to guard carefully against athletic endeavors ever leading to this tragic state. Consequently, our guidelines are reached always in response to the following question: "What would the athlete be left with in the way of vision, if he lost the vision in his best eye as a result of a sports injury?" The chart, to follow later in *Item IV*, will reflect this philosophy, and the phrase therein, "loss of function of one eye," means lack of visual correctibility to 20:80 or better.

Football players, who would not be able to participate without some form of visual correction because of the magnitude or type of their necessary correction factor, should be required to use contact lenses, which are all made of unbreakable and unshatterable plastics. Frame glasses ("spectacles") should not be allowed in this 'collision' sport because of their potential for conversion into a weapon for eye injury when dislodged.

Unbreakable and shatter-proof lenses and sturdy 'athletic' frames (those designed and manufactured specifically for use in vigorous sports), should be required for all eyeglass-wearing athletes in contact sports other than football, unless they also choose to use contact lenses.

Once again, the athlete in the special category of having "only one good eye," deserves special mention here with respect to contact sports. From football and ice hockey, he should be permanently disqualified. For the other contact sports, if he (or she) normally wears glasses in sports activities, then it should be required that they are of the 'athletic' frame with safety lenses variety, as described in the preceding paragraph. Contact lenses are not ideal protection for the "glasses-wearing" eyes in contact sports other than football, wherein the helmet and face-mask provide the primary protective barrier, and they should not be acceptable protection in contact sports for the monocular-vision athlete. For the "only-one-good-eye" athlete who does not ordinarily wear any glasses (and this is often the case actually); the use of a plane (no correction factor), safety-lens, "athletic"-frame pair of spectacles as a protective shield to his, or her, "one good eye" in non-football contact sports, is indicated and vigorously urged. The same protective use of 'plane' safety glasses (as described herein) is also in order in small-ball, non-contact sports, such as tennis, squash, hand-ball, paddle-ball (exception, golf).

F. Ears – An externally-worn hearing aid should not

be worn in contact sports because it, also, represents a potential weapon for causing injury itself; and therefore, the athlete who is significantly deaf overall should be restricted from contact sports. This restriction in view of his inability to respond to team signals and to the officials' controlling directives. Unilateral deafness probably would not preclude participation in contact sports unless associated with acute or chronic infection. Previous radical mastoid surgery would probably have rendered the skull sufficiently thin in the surgical area to make subsequent contact sports unwise; however, such post-surgical cases are becoming increasingly more infrequent in this antibiotic era.

G. *Respiratory* – Since efficient respiratory function is so much synonomous with good athletic performance, it is pertinent to enumerate the listed (see below and in *Item IV*) potentially disqualifying respiratory conditions in addition to acute infections (see Item III A. above). "Significant pulmonary insufficiency" might refer to emphysema, bronchiectasis, or cystic fibrosis, or to a combination of these, or to other more rare pulmonary problems. Spontaneous pneumothorax (unilateral) should be restricted from contact and endurance sports for a period of 3 months following full re-expansion of the effected lung; whereas, bilateral or recurrent pneumothorax would most likely preclude any further competition in either of these sports categories for at least one year (12 months). The relatively new approach to Tuberculosis therapy referred to as "INH Chemoprophylaxis," should not be considered disqualifying provided the student athlete is clinically well and is considered as an 'inactive' TB case.

H. *Cardiovascular* – Perhaps no other area of the medical history and examination is more important than the cardiovascular system. For there are non-pathological heart murmurs, mild situational ("exam-room anxiety") blood pressure elevations, and transient physiological pulse irregularities; none of which should limit athletic participation. And, in like manner, there may be significant past and/or present cardiovascular problems which only a thorough, current medical history and examination will bring to clarity, and which will have a direct and vital bearing on the candidate's qualifications for various sports. The only way to arrive at the proper decision for the student in question is a full and considerate evaluation of all factors, using consultants where and when indicated.

19

Generally speaking, valvular and/or cyanotic heart disease which have not required surgery prior to secondary school days, previously operated hearts (including the great vessels in the chest), organic hypertension (including coarctation of the aorta), active carditis (of any type) currently or within 3 previous months, significant pulse irregularities, and thrombo-embolic cardiovascular disease; are all sufficient cause for restricting both contact and endurance types of sports participation. Noteworthy exceptions to these general restrictions might be: a) a successfully surgically-repaired, and subsequently asymptomatic, patent ductus arteriosus, and b) acute superficial and/or deep thrombophlebitis; both of which should probably be only temporarily disqualifying in the same manner as an acute illness or injury.

I. Liver and Spleen – Sharp or blunt contusing injury to either of these organs can be a life-threatening event if said injury were to produce a tear in the organ capsule and subsequent intra-abdominal hemorrhage. Consequently, the pathologically enlarged liver and/or spleen, with the increased tension and fragility of its capsule, should preclude both contact and endurance sports. However, not infrequently, in young people with lean, slender, athletic bodies, either the liver or spleen may be palpable without evidence of any disease of the organ involved per se, or of any other systemic pathological condition. These cases are certainly qualified for endurance sports, but should be allowed to engage in contact sports only after a second medical opinion, only with extra protective padding to the areas, and only in consideration of frequent re-evaluations by the physician-in-charge to ascertain any change in status which might herald the early phase of some disease process.

Jaundice in the age group covered by this CODE almost invariably signifies an acute viral infection of the liver, and thereby disqualifying for all sports participation until complete recovery has occurred and has been maintained for at least six (6) weeks. Nevertheless and in addition, jaundice from any remote or less common cause should be equally restrictive to sports participation.

J. Kidneys, Herniae and Genitalia – Congenital or surgical absence of one kidney, or of one testicle, should restrict the candidate from interscholastic contact sports, as per the reasoning expressed previously in the discussion of candidates with "only one eye." In addition, for boys, when evaluating a potential athlete's genitalia, since the function of sperm production is the vital consideration for the testicle, and since an atrophic or an undescended testicle do not produce viable sperm, either of these conditions will be considered the same as an absent testicle in determining the boy's medical qualifications for participation.

Acute and chronic kidney disease cover such conditions as glomerulonephritis (Bright's disease), nephrosis, pyelonephritis, and associated renal insufficiency (uremia), and are not consistent with significant exertion, sports or otherwise, in any form.

Scrotal hydrocele is usually associated with an apparent, or an occult, inguinal hernia and is therefore afforded like consideration. In order that a blow directly over a hernia, which during sports exertion might well contain a short segment of small bowel, not lead to a serious bowel resection, this CODE directs that contact sports should be restricted until herniae (inguinal or femoral) and scrotal hydroceles are surgically repaired and are anatomically 'solid' 3 months thereafter.

K. Musculo-Skeletal System – Almost every evaluation and judgment in this realm must be individualized by the physician after thorough consideration of the condition under debate, the potential athlete as a whole, and the sport in question. Notwithstanding this fact of individualization of decision, however, some generalizations, and some specific guidelines, also, are in order and follow herewith.

Generally speaking, symptomatic structural abnormalities (congenital or acquired), acute or chronic inflammatory processes, and functional inadequacies (congenital or acquired) incompatible with the skill or contact demands of the sport in question, should all be reason enough for disqualifying the candidate until the condition has been thoroughly rectified, and until there seems little or no danger from reoccurrence and/or reaggravation by returning to participation. The vast majority of previous injuries to limbs and their joints will be judged for qualification (initial or return) on the basis of this 'functional adequacy' clause, and on the basis of whether they remain asymptomatic under vigorous sport use.

Specifically, a) because of the frequency of their occurrence, b) because of the need for medically appropriate and uniform decisions in their handling, and c) as examples of how general concepts are to be applied to actual conditions in an area of the medical evaluation, it is worth mentioning the following conditions. A history of herniated nucleus pulposus ('ruptured disc') *above* the L4-5 level, and most especially in the cervical area, should not be a candidate for contact sports because of the danger of and from reoccurrence therein. Spondylolisthesis (L5-S1 'slippage'), previous spinal surgery above the L4-5 level, and previous bony injury (fracture and/or dislocation) to the cervical spine, should all be disqualifying for contact sports on the basis of the real probability of aggravation and permanent damage via further major stress. In contrast, spina bifida occulta, lumbar spondylolysis, and 'old' disc at the L4-5 and L5-S1 areas (including remote surgical excision with or without fusion), would all be qualified, or not, primarily on the basis of current symptomatology.

Occasionally, the examining physician will encounter a candidate in whom an orthopedic surgeon has employed a device, usually metallic, to repair or facilitate healing of a fractured or diseased long bone. If said device is an actual joint prosthesis, then the candidate should be restricted from all but the most "leisure sports," and even then only after strict consideration of the general factors mentioned above. Candidates with intramedullary rods and those with plates and screws, would most likely not be qualified for either contact or endurance sports, although there might well be certain exceptions here. However, candidates in whom screws alone were used by the surgeon, would most likely be qualified for all sports; but not without emphasizing once again the need to consider first the symptoms-free and functional adequacy factors of the healed state.

L. Neurological System – In this section, we are discussing only the brain and associated intracranial structures, whose importance warrant consideration by themselves. The other components of the neurological system (spinal cord and peripheral nerves) are covered best in the physician's functional evaluation of the structures which they innervate, the musculoskeletal system.

Previous or current conditions which have left, or which are likely to have left, the brain and/or meninges scarred or dysfunctional; such as vascular accidents, surgery, infection, congenital abnormalities, malignancy, or trauma; should be considered disqualifying for all contact sports, and only considered qualified for endurance sports after careful deliberation of all factors. In this group would be found such not uncommon entities as sub-dural hematoma, epidural and sub-arachnoid hemorrhage, depressed skull fracture with or without laceration of brain substance, 'berry' aneurysm, hydrocephalus, and other less common clinical states.

Regarding cerebral concussions, this CODE utilizes the classification of the "Standard Nomenclature of Athletic Injuries (SNAI)" of the American Medical Association's Committee on the Medical Aspects of Sports, published in 1966, wherein the following differentiations are made:

CEREBRAL CONCUSSION, ACUTE, 1ST DEGREE (MILD)

symptoms: No loss of consciousness; variable symptoms of temporary memory impairment, mental confusion, unsteadiness, tinnitus, and/or dizziness.

signs: Perhaps none; or, appearance of brief period of mental confusion.

CEREBRAL CONCUSSION, ACUTE, 2ND DEGREE
(MODERATE)

symptoms: Transitory unconsciousness (up to 5 minutes) with retrograde amnesia; variable symptoms of mental confusion, tinnitus and headache.

signs: Appearance of transitory unconscious state and subsequent mental confusion.

CEREBRAL CONCUSSION, ACUTE, 3RD DEGREE (SEVERE)

symptoms: Unconsciousness for prolonged interval (more than 5 minutes) with prolonged period of retrograde amnesia; variable symptoms, but of greater duration than that experienced in mild or moderate types; possible convulsions.

signs: Appearance of prolonged unconscious state and subsequent mental confusion.

Taking our cue from the general consensus of experienced men in athletic medicine throughout the country, we conclude that the athlete who has sustained three or more 2nd or 3rd degree cerebral concussions in his previous lifetime has reached the point of dangerously increasing susceptibility to subsequent similar responses to lessening degrees of head trauma (like the 'glass-jawed' or 'punch-drunk' boxer), and therefore, should be excluded from further contact sports regardless of the protective equipment used.

Regarding convulsive disorders and athletics, it is essential first to have an accurate diagnosis from a qualified consultant in all such cases. Jacksonian epileptics should not be qualified for contact or endurance sports in that such a condition often signifies focal intracranial disease, as noted above ("brain and/or meninges scarred or dysfunctional"). Petit mal and psychomotor epilepsy, while in their active phases and/or under treatment, ordinarily cannot be sufficiently well controlled medically to allow for contact or endurance sports participation. If the condition here in petit mal and psychomotor forms is no longer active, and if no seizures have occurred for two treatment-free years, then certainly reconsideration for competitive athletics would be in order. Grand mal epileptics, however, are more predictable in their response to medical control, and if said treatment results in them having been seizure-free for at least two years immediately prior to their evaluation for interscholastic athletics, then we would find said candidates fully qualified contingent upon continued full seizure-control. In these cases, it is imperative that the appropriate coach be appraised of the neurological background of said specific athlete.

M. Other Medical Conditions – Certainly, there are additional rare and unusual conditions not covered in the foregoing discussions. Most often in these cases the physician's decision for sports qualification, or not, will not be a difficult one, and the course of appropriate action will be quite obvious; as it would be in the case of an active malignancy, or in cases of Cerebral Palsy, Muscular Dystrophy, Myasthenia Gravis, Multiple Sclerosis, or Addison's disease. However, occasionally the decision will be less clear, as it might be in cases of Graves' Disease, Regional Ileitis, Ulcerative Colitis, or certain neuropsychiatric problems; and then the decision must be left to the physician-in-charge, with the urging once more that he keep in mind the potentially beneficial effects of athletics, not just the well-publicized possible hazards.

N. Special Considerations – As part of this CODE, there are several peripheral considerations which need to be expressed and briefly discussed. Some of these matters, which follow, will be rather definitive rules, others will be guidelines of strong urging, and others will be hopefully helpful suggestions based on personal convictions. In this regard, where each matter fits should be obvious from the wording.

1. *Dental mouthpieces* – Following the lead of the National Federation of State High School Athletic Associations (NFSHSAA), mouthpieces should be required equipment for all interscholastic football players. They have been conclusively shown to significantly reduce dental injuries, soft tissue injuries of the face and mouth,

and cerebral concussions. The most effective type of mouthpiece is the custom-made (by a dentist) style for the upper jaw.

2. *Drugs, Alcohol, and Tobacco* — The non-medical use of sedatives, tranquilizers, or stimulants, or the use of narcotics or hallucinogens, ought to lead directly to dismissal from any and all interscholastic teams for the student, or students so involved. Team rules regarding the use of alcohol and tobacco are each coach's prerogative to set as he sees fit; yet the medical committee authorship of this CODE strongly supports those coaches whose decision is to forbid the use of said alcohol and tobacco among their athletes.

3. *Insurance* — That interscholastic athletic participants are totally uninsured, or inadequately insured, seems unrealistic in 1969; but this is. the case in a frighteningly significant percentage of said athletes. And although compulsory accident and injury insurance coverage for all participants in all interscholastic sports is an administrative, not medical, decision, it is endorsed here as a potential stimulus to its actuality.

4. *Medical Coverage* — This much-traveled and much-abused term can refer to an almost endless spectrum of actual circumstances depending upon local customs. This spectrum of meaning will include: a doctor and/or athletic trainer on the field, a school nurse in her office, a coach with his background of a couple of courses in health and athletic injuries during his college days plus the practical experience of his coaching years, an ambulance with its First Aid Team in the area, or a doctor in his office some variable distance removed from the sports area and yet aware of the fact that practice or a game is going on, and that he is providing the "medical coverage" (that he might be needed and called quickly to the sports area). This CODE contends that said "medical coverage" can only be provided in its true sense by a physician, and that only he (or she) can delegate the authority to someone else. Furthermore, it is strongly urged that all schools with organized interscholastic athletic programs have a responsible and committed athletic medicine advisor (who will be a physician), whose duty it should be to keep informed of *all* sports practices and at-home competition schedules within his school. For said sports practices and competitions, he will sometimes be present in person, and at other times he will stand ready to respond immediately if needed to the place summoned by his personally appointed on-the-scene representative (trainer, nurse,

coach, or other). For all 'home' contests of his particular school in football and ice hockey, the advisor in athletic medicine ought to be present himself. In case of unavoidable unavailability for any of the aforementioned responsibilities, said advisor should arrange for a responsible substitute and should inform all concerned. Treatment of athletic injuries other than that of an immediate nature rendered by the "medical coverage" of practices and contests, is not within the province of this CODE, and should be handled according to local and regional medical and school policies.

5. *Primacy of Medical Decisions* — Paramount to all that has been thus far expressed, ought to be the understanding that medical decisions should be respected and adhered to without being contested or resisted. It is the physician's responsibility to render an honest and compassionate medical judgment, with willing explanations when requested, to the best of his ability, considering all factors and all interested parties to the decision; – and it will be the coach's, the school's, the student's, and his (or her) parents' joint responsibility to accept said judgment without argument. This CODE intends, as one of its most important functions, to create the climate for both sides to this mutual responsibility.

6. *Immunizations* — It should be mandatory for every student interscholastic athlete to have a current, protectively-immunized status to tetanus and to poliomyelitis (oral Sabin-type vaccine) as part of his (or her) preseason medical evaluation. Hypersensitivity status to the immunizing biological product, or valid religious objections to the use of same, must be decided individually by the physician on the basis of the relative hazards involved.

ITEM IV – TABULAR EXPRESSION OF MATERIAL
DISCUSSED IN ITEM III

TABLE 1

Systems & Conditions	SPORTS Contact Endurance Leisure (x — recommended disqualification)		
A. Comparative immaturity (see football minimums)	x		
B. Acute infections	x	x	x
C. Blood and related conditions hemophilia and other bleeding tendencies	x		
anemia	x	x	
leukemia-lymphoma group	x	x	
D. Diabetes mellitus, inadequately controlled	x	x	

26

E. Eyes (see text re: contact lenses and 'safety' glasses)			
absence or loss of function of one eye	x		
severe myopia, even if correctible	x		
detached retina, even if surgically repaired	x		
F. Ears			
significant bilateral hearing loss (deafness)	x		
previous radical mastoid surgery	x		
G. Respiratory			
Tuberculosis, active and/or under ment	x	x	x
significant pulmonary insufficiency	x	x	
asthma, inadequately controlled	x	x	
H. Cardiovascular			
valvular and cyanotic ht. dis., recent carditis	x	x	x
previous heart or great-vessel surgery, organic hypertension, significant pulse irregularity, thrombo-embolic C-V disease	x	x	
I. Liver and Spleen			
jaundice, whatever cause	x	x	x
palpable liver and/or spleen			
pathological enlargement	x	x	
'postural' palpability (see text)	?		
J. Kidneys			
acute or chronic disease (functional insufficiency)	x	x	x
unilateral absence	x		
Herniae (inguinal and femoral) and Hydrocele	x	x	
Genitalia – absent, undescended, or atrophic testicle, unilateral	x		
K. Musculo-Skeletal (see examples in text: Item III K.)			
symptomatic structural abnormalities	x	x	x
inflammatory processes	x	x	x
functional inadequacies	x	x	x
Orthopedic surgical devices (metallic)			
intra-medullary rods	x	x	
plates and screws	x	x	
screws only	none		
prosthetic joints	x	x	x
L. Neurological (see text for discussion: Item III L.)			
conditions of brain-meningeal scarring and/or dysfunction (ex.: vascular accidents, surgery, concussions)	x		
certain convulsive disorders (see text)	x	x	

M. Other various medical conditions (see text)	case-individualized decisions
N. Special considerations: dental mouthpieces, drugs-alcohol-tobacco, insurance, "medical coverage," primacy of medical decisions and immunizations (see preceding text).	

ITEM V – CODE IMPLEMENTATION, CHANGE, AND MEDICAL-DECISION REVIEW

A. *Implementation* – The responsibility for the distribution of this CODE, and any subsequent modifications of it, to Maine secondary schools with interscholastic athletic programs, will be cooperatively shared by the Maine State Principals' Association and the Maine State Coaches' Association. As continually stressed in all foregoing sections, the intent of this CODE is to set forward recommended guidelines having to do with the medical aspects of conducting an interscholastic athletic program; and that these guidelines will have statewide uniformity and will be based upon the endorsed values of fitness, health education, competition and safety. That this CODE will be *the* adopted set of guidelines for each Maine secondary school in their sports program can be no more strongly urged than by appealing to the universal virtues of "good sportsmanship" and "same rules for all."

In like manner, the Committee on the Medical Aspects of Sports of the Maine Medical Association will be responsible for maintaining an up-dated version of the CODE with all practicing physicians (M.D. and D.O.) in the State, and for promoting the attitude of physician adherence to the CODE in decisions concerning interscholastic athletic medicine.

B. *Change* – It is only prudent to recognize from the outset that ours is a changing culture and a changing world; that we will see changes in medical treatment and technology, changes in athletic rules, equipment and techniques, and changes in social attitudes towards sports. Some of these changes will undoubtedly necessitate modifications (additions, deletions, or re-structures) in this CODE; and provision for same, under the combined endorsement of the responsible educational and medical leadership (see Item V A., above) is herewith authorized.

C. *Medical-Decision Review* – All the rules and guidelines herein presented are not precise and absolute pro and con, and all indecisions cannot be resolved by changing said rules as per the preceding section. Many medical decisions for qualification, or conversely for disqualification, as has been repeatedly emphasized throughout the foregoing body of this CODE, involve relative and circumstantial matters, and must be individualized with a workable solution being delivered by the physician on the case in question. Even so, an occasional (and hopefully rare) situation will arise where the decision seems locally insoluble, and provision is herewith made for a State Review Panel to settle said indecisions. This Review Panel will consist of one member from the Maine State Principals' Association, one member from the Maine State Coaches' Association, and one member from the Sports Medicine Committee of the Maine Medical Association. Cases devoid of local decision will only be considered when submitted jointly by the responsible local medical and educational authorities. The Review Panel will not function to substitute for local work and understanding, nor will it function to settle local personal disputes.

ITEM VI – SOURCE MATERIAL FOR CODE

1. "A Guide for Medical Evaluation of Candidates for School Sports" – Second Edition (1968) – Committee on the Medical Aspects of Sports, American Medical Association.
2. "Standard Nomenclature of Athletic Injuries" – 1966 – Committee on the Medical Aspects of Sports, American Medical Association.
3. "Medical Policy in Athletics" from the Staff Manual of the Department of Physical Education and Athletics, University of Maine (Orono) – in publication.
4. "Recommended Standards and Practices for a College Health Program" – 1964 – American College Health Association.
5. "Guide for Interscholastic Athletic Disqualification" – January 18, 1968 – Wisconsin Interscholastic Athletic Association.
6. Medical history and physical examination record forms; student participation, parental consent form – National Federation of State High School Athletic Associations.
7. "Desirable Athletic Competition for Children of Elementary School Age" – 1968 – American Asso-

ciation of Health, Physical Education and Recreation
– Washington, D.C.

8. "Minimum Standards of Physical Fitness Required of Candidates for Collision Sports at the University of Maine," J. D. Clement, Jr., M.D., et al – The Journal of the Maine Medical Association, 58:121 (June 1967).
9. "Accident Prevention Research in Sports," Kenneth S. Clarke, Ph.D. – Journ. AAHPER, Vol. 40: No. 2, p. 45 (February 1969).
10. "The High School Team Physician" – Robert E. Reibeld, M.D. – Proc. 7th National Conf. Med. Aspects of Sports (AMA-1965) – pg. 50.
11. "Philosophy and Standards for Girls' and Women's Sports" – DGWS-AAHPER – Washington, D.C. – 1969.

An international research program for the standardization of physical fitness tests

by

LEONARD A. LARSON

This century will be recorded in history as an age of great advancements in science and technology. Many developments since 1900 have a direct relationship to the health and fitness of the people. Some developments are favorable (advances in knowledges and skills in science and medicine) and some are unfavorable (lack of physical work and exercise in daily tasks and living practices that tend to lower the levels of health and fitness). In most cases, due to the lack of physical and medical examinations and particularly standards, the people are unaware of their "state of health and fitness". And, in nearly all cases, the people do not understand the long-ranged effects of many daily practices that ultimately will have damaging results.

At the ICSS (International Congress of Sport Sciences) conference in Tokyo in 1964 (during the Olympic Games) a first session was held on the problem of health and fitness of people internationally. A committee on the Standardization of Physical Fitness Tests (ICSPFT) was appointed and requested to set standards and to construct instruments for the measurement of physical fitness. The tentative plans were approved by the Executive Committee of ICSS at the closing session of the conference in 1964. Work was then begun in preparation of the research program to be reviewed, a year following, in Tokyo. This report deals with plans resulting from the 1965 meetings.

Objectives

The objectives were formulated at the 1964 conference and reaffirmed at the 1965 meeting. The motivation, in long range, is to provide the scientific instruments to study and to determine the powers and the organic resources of the people living under greatly varying conditions over the world. It was agreed that the first task is one of instrumentation and standards. In order that results can be made comparable, the test items and examination procedures need to be established and standardized.

To give specific direction for the work of the research committee, the following objectives were prepared and approved.

1. International survey of tests, measurements, and instruments for the determination of the physical fitness (abilities) of the human organism;

2. Identification, measurement and validation of procedures for the determination of the physical fitness of the or-

ganism related to sustained physical work and strenuous sports activity;

3. Standardization of the medical examination prerequisite to sustained physical work and sports activity involving all related systems, functions and organs of the body.

Research Program

The research program was planned in 1964 with some additions made in 1965. Procedures on the implementation of the program were also developed. It is the unanimous opinion of the committee that time and effort is now to be placed on research—not planning, except for minor adjustments. The committee represents a working research group. The most important qualification is an agreement to assume a share in the research program. Each committee member will, by interests and qualifications, be working on one or two phases of the program. It is expected that when interests are expressed, that each member will probably concentrate on one phase of the work.

Part I: The Survey. It was agreed in 1964 that an international survey be conducted on tests, measurements and instruments applied for the determination of the physical fitness in various countries throughout the world. Dr. Ishiko, Chairman of the Executive Committee, was placed in charge of this work. Some of the findings were reported at the 1965 meetings.

The survey includes tests, achievement standards and procedures for test administration. The survey also reports the measurement objectives (various phases of fitness and abilities), test items, re-

33

liabilities, validity and procedures for determinations, norms and methods of construction. The survey is continuing for more complete results. The central office for analysis and records is in Tokyo.

Part II: The Program. The basic research program can be classified as Performance Tests of Physical Fitness (6 phases), the work capacity tests (physiological), the medical examination and measurements of physique and body composition. All phases represent important aspects of physical fitness when estimated by sustained physical work or physical activity.

Agreements were reached on the basic constituents of the total research program. The elements and definitions represent guides in each phase. Establishing direction toward the objectives of standardizing physical fitness is of major significance, particularly when work will be accomplished in a number of laboratories.

1. Muscular strength (ability to exert muscular force against resistance).

2. Speed (ability to sustain action of power with maximal effort).

3. Muscular power (ability to mobilize muscular resources in one concentrated effort).

4. Muscular endurance (ability to sustain muscular action).

5. General endurance (ability to sustain action involving functions of respiration and circulation).

6. Organic integration of physical resources (ability to integrate physical movements).

7. Work Capacity (ability of the organic systems of the body to sustain the stresses of physical work).

8. Medical examinations (ability of the organism to sustain and favorably react to physical and emotional work stresses).

9. Physique, body composition (structural composition and body proportions).

It was agreed that the medical examinations should include all organic systems which are related to sustained physical work. This should include both effects and affects. Evidence on some phases appear to give significance to particular research, however, the elements that seem to have some importance will be included. They are:

1. Integumentary system.
2. Nervous system.
3. Muscular system.
4. Skeletal system.
5. Endocrine system.
6. Respiratory system.
7. Cardiovascular system.
8. Digestive system.
9. Genito-urinary system.
10. Nutritive system.
11. Metabolic system.
12. Reproductive system.
13. Sensory system.
14. Glandular system.

Part III: Sampling Factors. In looking ahead to the applications of the tests, a session was held on sampling conditions and procedures. These are now in the process of evaluation. Some change is likely.

It is the opinion of the research committee that race and ethnic factors, including age and sex, are significant sampling qualities. Recognizing the wide range of physical environmental conditions, in the various countries, climate, nutrition, altitude and air pollution are also of high significance. Personal elements include habitual physical activity and chronic diseases.

The design for the measurement of each factor will be determined at a later time —probably at the 1966 meeting.

Part IV : Applications. A study of the health and physical fitness status of the people, in many countries, is the ultimate purpose of the research work. It is recognized in world athletic competition that large differences are found among young participants. It is the desire of the committee to collect data that will more precisely describe the differences. It will then be possible to correlate the conditions of living to establish cultural variables that are significantly related to the health and fitness of the people.

A great need exists in the world for knowledge and help toward developing a physically strong organism. Systematic determinations will aid in noting the changes as the result of improved hygiene and ways of life. The most cherished result will be the improvement in general health as the result of improving the physical resources for each individual.

How To Prevent Heat Stroke In Football Players

Anderson Spickard, M.D. *and* Joe Worden

Heat stroke is a serious form of heat illness which results in a significant number of deaths in athletes. Football players who are not acclimatized to the heat or the vigorous demands of football practice are particularly vulnerable to this catastrophe. Under the present rules of the NCAA, college coaches and trainers have approximately three weeks to condition their players before the first game. In that brief period, players must become physically fit and mentally trained to carry out their position assignments. If the weather is hot during this strenuous period and proper precautions not taken, serious heat illness and even fatal heat stroke may occur.

Prevention of heat stroke is now possible. A technique has been devised in the Armed Forces to predict hazardous heat conditions during physical training exercises. Here, we will review this technique now in use at Vanderbilt University. Another method, currently used by other teams for prevention of heat illness in their players, will also be described.

Heat cramps and heat exhaustion are mild forms of heat illness and may precede the fully developed picture of heat stroke. Heat cramps are painful spasms of the calf and thigh muscles relieved by rest and extra salt intake.

The symptoms of heat exhaustion are similar to those of heat stroke, namely giddiness, weakness and nausea. Rest and replacement of salt and water is usually sufficient therapy for this condition.

Heat stroke, the severest form of heat illness, is a medical emergency. Diagnosis and treatment must be given promptly or irreversible changes in vital organs or even death occurs. A player who suffers from early symptoms of heat stroke complains of giddiness and nausea. Occasionally he notices an inability to cool off completely after a very hot practice. Usually he has lost considerable weight during the practice. He may collapse and when examined is unconscious, has hot dry skin, a fast pulse and rapid rate of respiration. His oral temperature may be elevated to 108°F or 110°F. If a player develops this condition, the uniform should be removed and the body cooled with towels soaked in ice water. Additional therapy includes replacement of salt and water which is best accomplished with intravenous salt solutions given under the direction of a physician.

The number of heat stroke fatalities in football players seems to be increasing. In the period 1933-1963, 15 players died from heat stroke; in the three year period 1963-1966, 11 players succumbed to this illness.[1] Many players have been ill with heat stroke each year, but the prevalence of the non-fatal illness is not known.

We have reviewed the previous cases of heat stroke to determine possible causes and ways to prevent them. From this review we have made the following observations:

First, heat stroke cases occur most often in the

first week of football practice. Of nine fatalities in high school football from 1953 to 1963, five occurred on the first day of practice and two on the second day. The remaining two occurred later in the week.[2]

Second, the value of heat acclimatization is not recognized by coaches and trainers. A player may be physically fit for practice in cool weather but very susceptible to heat illness if the weather is hot and humid. Studies on military personnel during World War II, have shown the 10 to 14 days are necessary for complete heat acclimatization.[3] The function of the heart, kidneys and other vital organs undergo profound alterations in hot weather and must be conditioned slowly to function efficiently in the heat. For example, studies have demonstrated that a heat acclimatized individual loses less salt in the sweat and will require less salt tablets to maintain adequate salt content in the body than an unacclimatized person.[3] The stress imposed by excessive heat and the physical demands of a football practice can be such that the unacclimatized person cannot lose heat effectively because of inefficient sweat glands.

Third, football uniforms are heavy and restrict evaporation of sweat. Sweating is the body's most efficient means of heat elimination.

Fourth, players are anxious to please coaches and are reluctant to report early symptoms of heat illness. Many authorities believe that heat stroke begins with the earlier symptoms of heat cramps or heat exhaustion and can be prevented if salt and water replacement is instituted early and adequate rest provided. Players must be encouraged to report danger signs of heat illness in themselves or their fellow players.

Fifth, many coaches and trainers incorrectly believe that the only way to prevent heat stroke is to take enough salt tablets. Although salt and water depletion contributes to the development of heat stroke, this is not the major factor. Heat stroke occurs when the player cannot lose heat into a hot and humid atmosphere.

Therefore, the most important part of any program of heat illness prevention is the determination of dangerous levels of heat and humidity. The technique used by the Army and Marines to measure these dangerous levels is now available and can be easily adapted for use by football teams.

A Heat Index (HI) is calculated twice in each practice. Practice routines are then altered if the HI is in the danger zone. The HI is calculated from three thermometer readings: a wet bulb thermometer, a dry bulb thermometer and a black globe thermometer (Figures 1 & 2). The wet bulb is a thermometer attached to a wick in water. The temperature recorded by this thermometer depends on the moisture content of the air. A low moisture content permits evaporation from the wick which low-

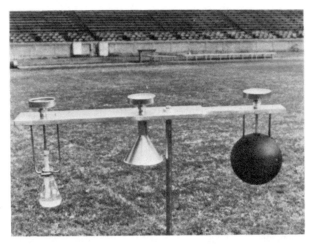

FIGURE 1—Heat Index (TI) thermometers. On the left is the wet bulb thermometer, in the middle the dry bulb thermometer, and on the right the black globe thermometer. (Published with permission of The Southern Medical Journal).

ers the wet bulb temperature. The dry bulb thermometer measures air temperature unaffected by moisture content. The black globe thermometer records heat from the rays of the sun. The HI is the sum of 70% of the wet bulb reading, plus 10% of the dry bulb reading, plus 20% of the black globe reading. A sample calculation of the HI

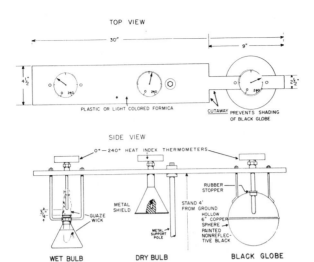

FIGURE 2—*Scale drawing of the Heat Index (HI) thermometers. The black globe is an ordinary industrial tank float ball painted a non reflective black. It can be purchased at any plumbing supplies store. (Published with permission of the Southern Medical Journal).*

is as follows:

Wet bulb reading	**75° x 0.7 =**	**52.5**
Dry Bulb reading	**88° x 0.1 =**	**8.8**
Black Globe reading	**111° x 0.2 =**	**22.2**
Heat Index		**83.5**

This is not an unusual HI on some days in late August or early September. In the Armed Forces when the HI is below 80, no precautions against heat illness are taken. Between HI readings of 80 and 85, training routines for unacclimatized recruits are lightened. When the HI is 85 or above, exercise by all recruits is prohibited.

The following adaptations of these procedures are recommended for use by football teams.

HI below 80 — No precautions against heat stroke are necessary.

HI 80 to 85 — Drills in full uniform should not be allowed during the first week of practice. Practice in shorts and T-shirts is preferred. After heat acclimatization is complete, limited drills in full uniforms can be conducted safely.

HI above 85 — All drills in full uniform are cancelled. If the HI is above 85 during the first week of practice, indoor sessions are preferred.

Other teams measure heat and humidity by use of a sling psychrometer (Figures 3A & 3B). This instrument measures only the wet bulb and dry bulb temperature. The relative humidity is read by matching these two temperatures on a scale. Practice procedures are altered according to the guidelines suggested by Dr. Murphy of Ohio State University.[4]

Wet Bulb Temperature	Precautions
Under 60° F	None necessary
61° to 65°F	Alert observations of all squad members, particularly those who lose considerable weight.
66° to 70°F	Insist that salt and water be given on field.
71F° to 75F°	Alter practice schedule to provide rest period to every 30 minutes in addition to above precautions.
76°F and Higher	Practice postponed or conducted in shorts.

(Whenever the relative humidity is 95% or higher, great precautions should be taken.)

In both the calculation of the HI and use of the sling psychrometer readings the wet bulb is considered the most important indicator of dangerous heat levels. The HI calculation includes an additional measurement of radiant heat (the black globe temperature). We prefer the HI method for this reason. Radiant heat can be substantial even on cloudy days and sufficient to elevate the HI above 80.

Other measures to prevent heat stroke include adequate replacement of salt and water. A player who loses 6.6 lbs. of weight after a practice perspires about a quart of water and the amount of salt in twenty-one 0.5 gram salt tablets. We have observed that most players tolerate this amount of

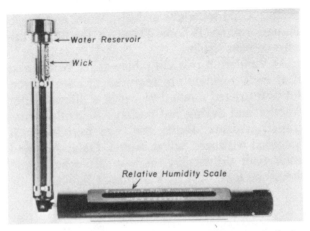

FIGURE 3A—Sling psychrometer. The wet and dry bulb thermometers are attached to the extended arm. The gauze wick of the wet bulb is moistened by a water reservoir. The arm with attached thermometers is twirled around to allow air movements to cool the wet bulb.

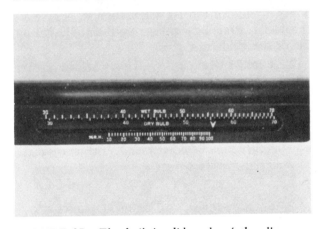

FIGURE 3B—The built-in slide rule of the sling psychrometer correlates wet and dry bulb thermometer readings to give relative humidity percentage. Bacharach Instrument Company, 200 N. Braddock Avenue, Pittsburgh, Pennsylvania, 15208. Catalog Code 12-2006.

water and salt loss without difficulty if the weather is cool. This is not true if the weather is hot. The player who loses over five pounds of weight after a practice in hot weather usually complains of

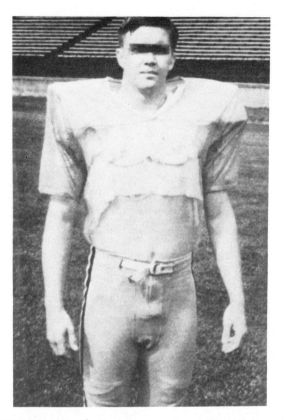

FIGURE 4—*Football player wearing nylon "fish-net"
jersey over shoulder pads and a shortened T-Shirt. The
large mesh allows proper heat loss from the body. The
jersey is tucked into the pants. (Published with permission
of the Southern Medical Journal).*

giddiness and weakness and his mental and physical performance is poor. These are the first symptoms of heat stroke.

At Vanderbilt two salt tablets taken before and after each practice are required of each player. An unrestricted amount of water is allowed after practice and during rest periods. Recently a new grapefruit drink, Wink, has been introduced. It is cooled with ice. Salt is added. Gater-Ade and other fruit drinks have a low salt content and should be used only as a source of liquid.

SUMMARY

Heat stroke in football players can be prevented

by use of the following procedures:

1. Football practice in hot weather should be conducted in the very early morning or late afternoon. Dangerous levels of heat should be determined by use of the HI calculation or sling psychrometer. Practice routines are then adjusted by use of the guidelines given.

2. Summer workouts by players before regular practice begins should be done in the sun when it is hot and humid. This will gradually begin the process of heat acclimatization.

3. Uniforms should be lightweight for players who practice in hot environments (Figures 4 & 5).

4. Coaches and trainers should observe their players for early symptoms and signs of heat illness especially the first week or ten days of practice. Players should be encouraged to report early symptoms of heat illness in themselves or fellow players.

5. Two or three 0.5 gram salt tablets before

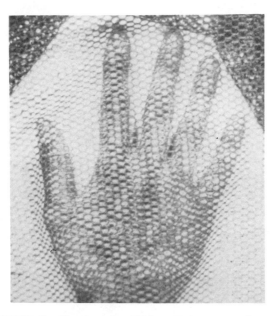

FIGURE 5—Hand under "fish-net" jersey to demonstrate size of mesh. (Published with permission of the Southern Medical Journal).

and after each practice should be required of each player. Frequent rest periods and as much water as a player needs to quench his thirst should be provided. Any player who loses over five pounds after a practice in the heat is a likely candidate to develop heat stroke and requires more rest, more salt and more water replacement than outlined above.

BIBLIOGRAPHY

1. Blyth, C. S. and Arnold, D. C.: **Thirty-Fifth Annual Survey of Football Fatalities 1931-1966.** Proceedings of the Forty-Fourth Annual Meeting. American Football Coaches Association, 1967.

2. Kaufman, W. S.: **The Effect of Football Equipment on Core Temperature, Heart Rate, Oxygen Uptake and Pulmonary Ventilation of Athletes,** Doctoral Dissertation, Ohio State University Graduate School, Columbus, Ohio, 1964.

3. Conn, J. W.: **The Gordon-Wilson Lecture—Some Clinical and Climatological Aspects of Aldosteronism in Man.** Trans. Amer. Clin. and Climat. Ass. 74:61-91, 1962.

4. Murphy, R. J. and Ashe, W. F.: **Prevention of Heat Illness in Football Players,** JAMA 194: 650-654, (Nov. 8), 1965.

Heat Stroke in College Football and Suggestions for Prevention

ANDERSON SPICKARD, M.D.

HEAT STROKE is a severe form of heat illness which may occur in persons who exercise in an excessively hot and humid environment. Victims of heat stroke collapse suddenly, usually become unconscious, and when examined are hyperthermic, hypotensive and have marked tachycardia and tachypnea. This is a serious emergency. Treatment must be started at once or irreversible damage to the brain, liver and kidneys may ensue. When heat stroke is accompanied by coma, a mortality of 22% has been reported.[1]

Fatal heat stroke in football players occurs annually and the number of such episodes is increasing. In a study of football deaths from

Supported in part by the John B. Howe Fund for Medical Research.

1931 to 1963 inclusive, 15 football players died of heat stroke, while in the 3 year period from 1963 to 1966 there were 11 football fatalities due to heat stroke.[2]

An understanding of the methods of prevention of heat stroke is, therefore, very important to football players, coaches and team physicians. At a recent conference on the medical aspects of sports, the importance of prevention of heat illness in football players was emphasized and a practical guide for procedures based on measurements of temperature and humidity on the practice field was outlined.[3]

The purpose of 'this paper is to report a case of heat stroke in a college football player, to discuss the environmental heat conditions under which the episode occurred and to present the method used by the Armed Forces to prevent similar catastrophes.

Case Report

A 19 year old white male student at Austin Peay College, Clarksville, Tenn., reported on Sept. 1, 1966, for his first day of football practice. At 5:40 P.M. he collapsed suddenly with heat stroke near the end of the second session on this first day of practice. During the summer he had worked at a very hot job on a factory assembly line. One month before reporting to practice he began training by running 2 to 4 miles each afternoon 5 days a week wearing shorts and a sweat shirt. A physician examined him the day before practice and found him to be fit. The morning practice lasted from 9:30 A.M. to 11:00 A.M. Players wore full uniforms consisting of white football pants, red jersey, full pads and a white helmet. The patient remembered that it seemed hard to get his breath. During the morning practice he lost 6 pounds, and he was too hot and tired to each lunch. He drank water and took 2 salt tablets.

The afternoon practice began at 3:30 P.M. and ended at 5:40 P.M. During the first hour, groups of players went through strenuous routines, such as "two on one," blocking drills on the sled, tackling and running dummy offensive plays. When he became ill, the patient was running up a hill 25 to 30 yards in length with other players. They ran up the hill 6 to 8 times and walked down. The patient stated that "I made it all the way, but on the last 5 times everything was blank. I collapsed after reaching the top on the eighth time." The coach described his appearance in the following way: "His eyes were sunken and pupils began to dilate. His breathing was labored. He was sweating,

48

his hands were cold, and he was completely motionless." He was taken to the Clarksville Hospital and within 10 minutes was being cooled by ice packs on the emergency room stretcher.

Physical examination revealed an unconscious man with a B.P. of 70/? mm. Hg. and a weak pulse. The pupils were constricted at first, then were dilated bilaterally. They remained reactive to light. Reflexes were hypoactive. He was perspiring. The initial rectal temperature was estimated at 110° F., (the thermometer registered only 108° F.). At 5:55 P.M., 5 minutes after he arrived in the emergency room, the temperature was 108° F. At 6:45 P.M., the rectal temperature was 104.8° F. and the B.P. 130/70 mm. Hg. By 7:05 P.M., the B.P. was 140/80 mm. Hg. and the T. 101.8° F. Medication at Clarksville included oxygen by nasal catheter, normal saline solution 1000 ml. intravenously, 5% dextrose in water 1000 ml. intravenously, metaraminol bitartrate (Aramine) intravenously, hydrocortisone (Solu-Cortef) 150 mg. intravenously, sodium secobarbital (Seconal) 130 mg. intravenously and chlorpromazine (Thorazine) 25 mg. intravenously. Jerking muscular contractions became very pronounced. Pharyngeal and tracheal secretions accumulated and suctioning was necessary.

He was transferred to Vanderbilt University Hospital at 8:00 P.M. that night, where examination revealed a B.P. of 94/70 mm. Hg., P. of 130 per minute and Kussmaul respiration at a rate of 30 to 40 per minute. The rectal temperature was 103° F. He was comatose and had a warm, dry skin. The neck was not stiff. The pupils were small, equal in size and reacted briskly to light. There was no papilledema. The deep tendon reflexes were active and equal. No Babinski or Hoffman signs were noted.

Laboratory data. W.B.C. count was 14,900 per cu. mm. with a normal differential except for an increased number of immature neutrophils. Hgb. was 15.7 Gm., PCV. 47%. Platelet count was 55,000 per cu. mm. The BUN. was 24 mg. per 100 ml., sodium 145, potassium 3.6, chloride 103 and bicarbonate 11 mEq./L.

He was immediately placed on a hypothermic blanket and the temperature reduced to below 100° F. He was given 5% dextrose in 0.5% saline solution 6000 ml. intravenously, and because of the possibility of cerebral edema dexamethazone (Decadron) intramuscularly to supplement the hydrocortisone he had received in Clarksville.

Six hours after admission he moved his head to spoken commands, but remained very lethargic. Three hours later he was oriented and could converse. On the 2nd hospital day he was much better and was fully awake without apparent neurologic abnormality. On this day there was laboratory evidence of renal and liver damage. The BUN. was 52 mg. per 100 ml., serum glutamic oxaloacetic transaminase (SGOT.) was 202 Karmen units, and prothrombin content 18%. On the 3rd hospital day the SGOT. was 870 Karmen units

49

and serum glutamic pyruvate transaminase (SGPT.) 415 Karmen units. Total bilirubin was 0.9 mg., BUN. 89 mg. and serum creatinine 6.2 mg. per 100 ml. Urine output was quite low initially (Fig. 1). The findings in the urine were compatible with acute renal damage.

After the first week diuresis occurred accompanied by a gradual decrease in the levels of the BUN. and creatinine (Fig. 1). Prothrombin and transaminase levels also indicated improved liver function. All elec-

FIG. 1

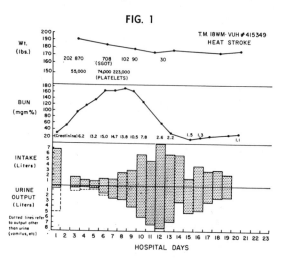

trocardiograms were normal. He was discharged after 3 weeks' hospitalization feeling well, and apparently suffering no deterioration in intellectual function.

Discussion

Football players and others exposed to excessive environmental heat can develop one or all of the three major clinical syndromes of heat illness. Heat cramps, the mildest of the three, are painful contractions of the calf muscles. These cramps result from excessive loss of sodium chloride in the sweat and can be prevented by generous replacement of salt in the diet, salt tablets or salt solutions. Heat exhaustion, a more severe form of salt depletion, produces pallor, weakness, sweating, muscle cramps and postural hypotension. Reduction in plasma volume is thought to be responsible for many of the symptoms which rapidly subside as saline solution is administered intravenously. Heat stroke described in this paper is the most severe of the three.

Prodromal symptoms of heat stroke may

warn of its onset and commonly include restlessness, mental confusion, nausea and headache.[4] Occasionally patients feel very hot and are unable to cool off completely. This was true in this patient.

The signs of heat stroke are predominately those related to alterations in the functions of the central nervous system and cardiovascular system. They include coma, delerium, convulsions and ataxia. Nuchal rigidity, decorticate posturing, hemiplegia, incontinence and flaccid muscles have been observed. Kussmaul respiration is usually present. Shock and tachycardia are frequent.[5]

Damage at the cellular level from heat stroke produces alterations in function of the kidneys, liver, myocardium, brain and hematopoietic system.[5-7] Ischemia of these organs resulting from shock accounts for some of the derangements of function. Various theories to explain the cellular damage from the hyperthermia itself have been proposed.[8]

Acute tubular necrosis was treated by careful fluid replacement during the oliguric and the diuretic phases (Fig. 1). Urinalysis and studies of renal function one year later have revealed no residual damage. Improvement in liver function accompanied the patient's general improvement and no abnormality was present one year later. Thrombocytopenia, anemia[5] and fibrinolysis[9] have been observed in victims of heat stroke. While the number of platelets in this patient was transiently diminished, no other hematologic disorder was present.

It is well to reemphasize the importance of reducing body temperature in the treatment of heat stroke. Austin and Berry[1] reported a mortality rate of 10% for patients whose recorded temperatures remained below 106° F. in contrast to 21% for those whose temperatures rose above this level. The rapid reduction in body temperature of the patient reported undoubtedly saved his life. Ten minutes after his collapse he was in the Clarksville Hospital emergency room. Five minutes later he was being cooled with ice packs and in one hour the temperature had been reduced approximately 8° F. Chlorpromazine as suggested by Hoagland[10] was used for its hypothermic effect and as a tranquilizer. Saline solutions intravenously were given rapidly to replace depleted salt and water. Oxygen by nasal catheter was used to treat anoxia associated with shock while metaraminol bitartrate (Aramine) intravenously supported the blood pressure until the plasma volume was restored.

The use of adrenocortical hormones in the treatment of heat stroke has been suggested by some observers.[11] The rationale for the use of this agent rests on the hypothesis that production of adrenal hormone is inadequate for the severe stress of heat stroke. They also reduce cerebral edema.[12] Malamud[5] has reported the presence of edema of all organs and particularly of the brain in persons dying of heat stroke. Undoubtedly, cerebral edema accounts for some of the signs of abnormal central nervous system function and it is important to reduce this edema as soon as possible.

Prevention of Heat Stroke in Football Players

There is no doubt that when heat stroke occurs an appraisal of the circumstances preceding the player's illness usually reveals that practice was unnecessarily strenuous, salt and water replacement was inadequate and rest periods infrequent. It is probable that in most instances of heat stroke light practice schedules, more rest periods and closer observations of the players for the appearance of prodromal symptoms would have prevented the final collapse. On the other hand, it has occurred in players when coaches and trainers have taken precautions which they considered adequate. The case reported here, and others like it, make it clear that there are many factors unique to football which make the prevention of heat stroke difficult.

(1) The environment is often very hot and humid in the late summer particularly in the

South as football practice begins all over the United States.

(2) Many players do not exercise during the summer and are not heat acclimatized when practice commences.

(3) Enthusiastic young players during the first days of strenuous exercise fear to admit they are exhausted, and do not report early symptoms of heat illness.

(4) Football uniforms are heavy and prevent proper heat elimination.

(5) Salt and water loss is great in football players and determination of replacement needs is difficult.

(6) Methods of objective measurement of environmental heat, although available, are not in general use by coaches and trainers.

Fatalities due to heat stroke in football occur during the first week of practice when the weather is hot and players are in poor physical condition. Of 9 fatalities in American high school football between 1956 and 1963, 5 occurred on the first day and 2 on the second day of practice. All were interior linemen.[13] Acclimatization to heat is very important in the prevention of heat stroke. Studies have shown that the rectal temperature of an acclimatized man is lower for a standard heat load and his heart rate is slower at a given temperature than the nonacclimatized.[14] Compensatory adjustment in the sweating mechanism, cardiovascular system and adrenocortical activity is more efficient in the heat acclimatized individual.[15,16] Approximately 10 to 20 days are required for complete heat acclimatization.[15]

The preseason workouts and the job in the factory were strenuous and probably resulted in some heat acclimatization in the patient reported here. It is difficult to understand why he collapsed while others probably less well conditioned did not. All players participated in the same exercises including the end of the practice "run up and down the hill." The patient had not been given extra drills. The uniforms of all players were identical. It appeared, therefore, that practice on that hot

FIG. 2

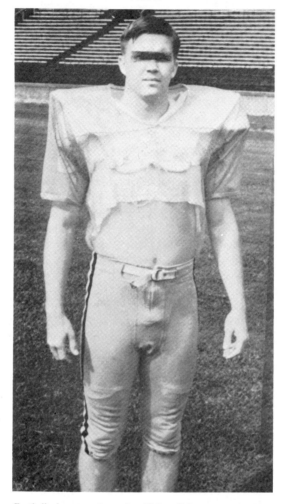

Football player wearing nylon "fish-net" jersey over shoulder pads and a shortened T-shirt for use in hot weather. The large mesh allows proper heat dissipation. The jersey may be tucked into pants as is a conventional jersey.

and humid day was more hazardous for this patient and in spite of strenuous preseason workouts he was inadequately acclimatized.

Practice on this first day was conducted in full football uniform. Kaufman[13] has shown, by measuring water loss, that work performed in football uniform is 70% more strenuous than the same work carried out in a hospital scrub suit. If it is excessively hot during the first week of practice, players should wear

FIG. 3

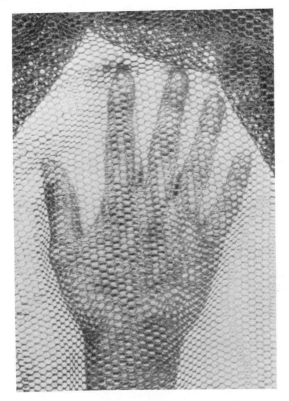

"Fish-net" jersey to demonstrate size of mesh.

shorts and T-shirts. If full uniforms and pads are worn, a "fish-net" jersey (Figs. 2 and 3) over a shortened T-shirt•permits dissipation of heat.

It is now recognized that adequate replacement of salt and water for those exercising in the heat is essential for prevention of heat illness. The limitation of water for athletes which was practiced years ago is known to have been a dangerous procedure. Weight loss during a practice session in the heat represents loss of salt and water. Murphy[3] emphasized the hazard of excessive weight loss and urged coaches and trainers to observe carefully players who lose 5 pounds or more during a practice in hot weather.

Scott[17] states that during light work heat is lost as follows: radiation, convection and conduction, 65%; evaporation of water from skin and lungs, 30%; warming of inspired air, 3%; excretion of urine and feces, 2 percent. Loss of body heat by radiation, convection and conduction ceases when environmental temperature and body temperature are the same. Evaporation of sweat is impaired when environmental humidity is high. Thus, 95% of the heat dissipating capacity of the body is impaired by high levels of temperature and humidity. Moreover, heat production is increased with heavy exercise. Heat stroke occurs more readily when this additional heat cannot be dissipated into the environment.

FIG. 4

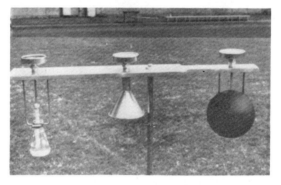

Heat Index (HI) thermometers. On the left is the wet bulb thermometer, in the middle the dry bulb thermometer and on the right the black globe thermometer.

It is essential that the technic used by the Army and Marine Corps to monitor the training of recruits in hot weather be understood and made available to football coaches and trainers. In these services, the amount of activity allowed recruits in hot weather depends on hourly measurements of three types of temperature: dry bulb temperature, wet bulb temperature and black globe temperature. To determine these temperatures, three thermometers are used as illustrated in figures 4 and 5. The first thermometer is a wet bulb thermometer. This thermometer is cooled by a gauze wick saturated with water. This read-

FIG. 5

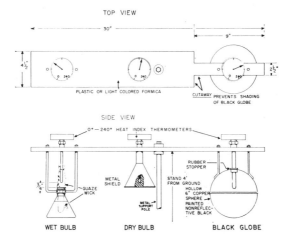

TOP VIEW

PLASTIC OR LIGHT COLORED FORMICA

CUTAWAY PREVENTS SHADING OF BLACK GLOBE

SIDE VIEW

0° — 240° HEAT INDEX THERMOMETERS

RUBBER STOPPER

METAL SHIELD

STAND 4' FROM GROUND

HOLLOW 6" COPPER SPHERE

PAINTED NONREFLEC- TIVE BLACK

GUAZE WICK

METAL SUPPORT POLE

WET BULB   DRY BULB   BLACK GLOBE

Scale drawing of the Heat Index (HI) thermometers.

ing is affected both by temperature and humidity and will always record a lower temperature than the dry bulb (the second thermometer) except when the humidity is 100 percent. At that time both temperatures are the same. The second thermometer is a dry bulb thermometer shielded from the direct rays of the sun. This reading is affected only by the air temperature. The third thermometer, the black globe thermometer, measures radiant heat or heat from the rays of the sun. The black globe thermometer consists of a 6 inch hollow copper sphere painted a nonreflective black and contains a thermometer with its bulb near the center. An index of environmental heat is calculated from the readings of these three thermometers. The index will be called the Heat Index (HI) and represents the sum of 70% of the temperature of the wet bulb plus 10% of the temperature of the dry bulb plus 20% of the temperature in the black globe. The use of three thermometers in calculating the HI gives a more comprehensive reading than can be obtained by the use of any of the thermometers alone. A sample calculation of the Heat Index is as follows:

The wet bulb reading is	75F×0.7=52.5
The dry bulb reading is	92F×0.1= 9.2
The black globe reading is	111F×0.2=22.2
Heat Index	83.9

This is not an unusual HI on a hot sunny day in late August.

The use of this index in training military recruits has resulted in a marked decrease in incidence of heat illness. No precautions against heat illness are taken when the HI is below 80. Between HI readings of 80 and 85, training routines for unacclimatized recruits are lightened. When the HI is 85 or above, exercise by all recruits is prohibited.[18,19]

The application of these standards to football is simple. When the HI is below 80, practice may proceed as scheduled. When the HI is between 80 and 85, practice in full uniform should be brief, and shorts and T-shirts preferred especially the first week or ten days of practice. Outside practice in full uniform should be cancelled when the HI is over 85.

In table 1 are listed the HI values recorded at Fort Campbell, Kentucky, a few miles from Austin Peay College on the day of the patient's illness. The highest HI values are in the afternoon hours on the day of illness. After 9:00 A.M. on that day the HI was over 80 except for one reading at 11 A.M. HI values are not available after 3:00 P.M. In retrospect, football practice with full uniform by young men who were not well conditioned to the heat was very hazardous both in the morning and the afternoon of the patient's illness.

The following suggestions are offered for the purpose of preventing heat stroke in football players.

Summer training should be encouraged to develop heat acclimatization. At least seven to ten days should be utilized for the development of heat acclimatization before strenuous practice in full uniform is allowed. Practice should be controlled as follows:

HI below 80—No precautions against heat stroke are necessary.

TABLE 1

SEPTEMBER 1, 1966

Time	Wet Bulb	Dry Bulb	Black Globe	Heat Index
7:00 AM	49.0	7.2	15.8	72.0
8:00 AM	50.4	7.8	18.0	76.2
9:00 AM	53.2	8.4	20.4	82.0
10:00 AM	51.1	8.7	20.2	80.0
11:00 AM	50.4	8.7	19.6	78.7
12:00 Noon	51.8	8.9	19.6	80.3
1:00 PM	52.5	9.0	21.0	82.5
2:00 PM	52.5	9.1	21.4	83.0
3:00 PM	51.8	9.1	20.4	81.3

Heat Index values on the day patient developed heat stroke.

The wet bulb value given is 70% the wet bulb temperature; dry bulb value 10% the dry bulb temperature; black globe value 20% the black globe temperature. The readings were made at Fort Campbell, Kentucky, a few miles from Austin Peay College.

HI 80 to 85—Drills in full uniform should not be allowed during the first week of practice. Practice in shorts and T-shirts is preferred. After heat acclimatization is complete, limited drills in full uniforms can be conducted safely.

HI above 85—All outdoor drills in full uniform should be cancelled.

Other supplemental measures are useful for prevention of heat stroke.

(1) Practice should be conducted in the early morning or late evening when the HI is usually low.

(2) Uniforms for practice should be light-weight.

(3) Adequate rest periods during practice and replacement of salt and water help to prevent heat stroke.

(4) Players who lose over 5 pounds during a practice session in hot weather or who fail to cool off completely between practices should be considered likely candidates for heat stroke.

The thermometers used in the calculation of the HI are easy to assemble and every team practicing in hot environments should have them on the field. The use of this objective measurement of environmental heat to limit football practice in hot weather, in addition to the application of the other preventive measures mentioned above, can prevent heat stroke in football players. If these preventive measures are not used, it can be predicted with certainty that one or more fatal cases of preventable heat stroke will occur annually among football players.

Acknowledgements. The author is grateful to Dr. Fount Russell, Clarksville, Tennessee, who referred the patient to Vanderbilt and to Mr. Walter Powers, Preventive Health Officer, Fort Campbell, Kentucky, who provided valuable assistance. Mr. Bailey Moore, Vanderbilt Hospital, constructed the HI thermometers.

References

1. Austin, M. D., and Berry, J. W.: Observations on One Hundred Cases of Heatstroke, JAMA 161:1525, 1956.
2. Blyth, C. S., and Arnold, D. C.: Thirty-Fifth Annual Survey of Football Fatalities 1931-1966. Proceedings of the Forty-Fourth Annual Meeting. American Football Coaches Association, 1967.
3. Murphy, R. J., and Ashe, W. F.: Prevention of Heat Illness in Football Players, JAMA 194:650, 1965.
4. Gottschalk, P. G., and Thomas, J. E.: Heat Stroke, Mayo Clin Proc 41:470, 1966.
5. Malamud, N., Haymaker, W., and Custer, R. P.: Heat Stroke—A Clinico-Pathologic Study of 125 Fatal Cases, Milit Surg 99:397, 1946.
6. Vesica, F. G., and Peck, O. C.: Liver Disease from Heat Stroke, Gastroenterology 43:340, 1962.
7. Ferris, E. B., Jr., Blankenhorn, M. A., Robinson, H. W., and Cullen, G. E.: Heat Stroke: Clinical and Chemical Observations on 44 Cases, J Clin Invest 17:249, 1938.
8. Burger, F. J., and Fuhrman, F. A.: Evidence of Injury to Tissues after Hyperthermia, Amer J Physiol 206:1062, 1964.
9. Meikle, A. W., and Graybill, R., Jr.: Fibrinolysis and Hemorrhage in a Fatal Case of Heat Stroke, New Eng J Med 276:911, 1967.
10. Hoagland, R. J., and Bishop, R. J., Jr.: A Physiologic Treatment of Heat Stroke, Amer J Med Sci 241:415, 1961.
11. Schillhammer, W. F., and Massonneau, R. L.: Heat Stroke: A Review of Three Cases, US Armed Forces Med J 9:1001, 1958.
12. Galicich, J. H., French, L. A., and Melby, J. C.: Use of Dexamethasone in Treatment of Cerebral Edema Associated with Brain Tumors, J Lancet 81:46, 1961.
13. Kaufman, W. S.: The Effect of Football Equipment on Core Temperature, Heart Rate, Oxygen Uptake and Pulmonary Ventilation of Athletes, Doctoral Dissertation, Ohio State University Graduate School, Columbus, Ohio, 1964.
14. Gila, T., Shibolet, S., and Sohar, E.: The Mechanism of Heat Stroke, J Trop Med Hyg 66:204, 1963.
15. Conn, J. W.: The Gordon-Wilson Lecture—Some Clinical and Climatological Aspects of Aldosteronism in Man, Trans Amer Clin Climat Ass 74:61, 1962.
16. Fox, R. H., Goldsmith, R., Hampton, I. F. G., and Lewis, H. E.: The Nature of the Increase in Sweating Capacity Produced by Heat Acclimatization, J Physiol 171:368, 1964.
17. Scott, J. W.: The Body Temperature, in Best, C. H., and Taylor, N. B.: *The Physiological Basis of Medical Practice: A Text in Applied Physiology.* Ed. 8, Baltimore, Williams and Wilkins Company, 1966, p. 1413.
18. Yaglou, C. P., and Minar, D.: Control of Heat Casualties at Military Training Centers, Arch Indust Health (Chicago) 16:302, 1957.
19. Prevention, Recognition and Treatment of Heat Casualties. U.S. Army Regulation No. 40-175, August 1, 1966. 101st Airborne Division and Fort Campbell, Kentucky.

Preseason Conditioning Exercises For High School Football Players

EDWARD D. HENDERSON, M.D.,
DONALD J. ERICKSON M.D.

MANY PHYSICIANS and coaches have long recognized the need for preseason conditioning before participation in competitive sports by both high school and college athletes as one means of reducing the incidence of injuries. The report by Honet and associates[1] showed that various aspects of physical fitness require several months of conditioning exercises for optimal development. Preconditioning was associated with an increase in maximal work output during the first two months of participation in high school football, whereas the control group (nonconditioned) showed a decline in maximal work output: results which indicated a need to reevaluate the effectiveness of the present system of training prior to the commencement of the football season. Other studies[2] have also shown that

---

*Published under the direction of the Committee on Medical Aspects of Sports of the Minnesota State Medical Association.

various aspects of physical fitness require at least several months of conditioning for optimal development.

Conflicting Rules

The National Federation of State High School Athletic Associations has recommended a period of several months of conditioning exercises prior to the onset of the athletic season.[1] However, this recommendation may be carried out in Minnesota only at the expense of violating the rules of the Minnesota State High School League as published in the official handbook:[3]

1. Practice may begin two (2) weeks prior to the first Monday in September.

2. Practice and the season will be terminated upon completion of the final game on the Official Schedule for each school.

3. No school may engage in any football game or games, practice, training or other football activities between the close of one season and the opening of the next season. . . . This regulation includes conditioning, training, or instruction conducted directly or indirectly by school officials or other interested individuals with the exception of the secondary students.

4. For practice sessions, the handbook states that two (2) weeks of organized practice ". . . must precede the first game. . . . nine (9) separate and complete days of practice must be held before school engages in interscholastic games." In addition: "Inter-school practice scrimmages may not be held until after five (5) separate and complete days of organized practice."

Therefore supervised or organized conditioning exercises prior to the opening date for practice would be considered a violation of the 1965-1966 rules of the Minnesota State High School League, and in apparent conflict[1] with the recommendations of the National Federation of State High School Associations, of which Minnesota is a member.

Preseason Program of Exercises

Addressing itself to this problem, the Committee on Sports Medicine of the Minnesota State Medical Association has formulated a program of exercises which is available to all high schools throughout the state. Thus, all the participants in competitive sports have an equal opportunity to undertake a program of preseason conditioning that will increase the level of physical fitness prior to the organized football practice in an effort to reduce the incidence of such injuries as are frequent in the early part of the season. However, it should be emphasized that physical fitness is only one of the factors that reduces the number of football injuries. Other factors are good coaching, proper equipment, adequate officiating, and good condition of the playing field.

A Physical Educator.

A careful search of the medical literature, as well as the literature in the field of physical education, failed to reveal a simplified program of progressive exercises for high school students without the need for uniforms or equipment. In the program of exercises to be presented, it is highly desirable that a trained leader, preferably a physical educator, lead the group on a regular basis so as to give continuity to the program as well as to ensure that the participants gradually increase the intensity of the exercises.

The exercises to be described are designed to improve the cardiovascular function, to strengthen muscles of the trunk and extremities, and to increase the flexibility of the body and legs. It is understood that once organized practice has begun, the coach will take over the program of exercises as part of the practice training.

Captain's Practice.

These exercises were presented to representatives of the Minnesota State High School League which went on record stating that this program

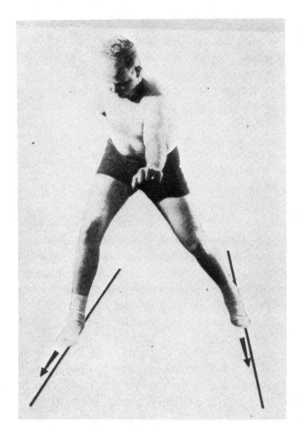

Figure 1

should be strongly encouraged. At the present time students in some high schools do participate in an informal and unsupervised program of preseason exercises known as "captain's practice." These groups of boys meet regularly and perform group exercises under a chosen leader, who may be the team captain.

These exercises should be performed in the order they are presented. The leader should determine the amount of exercise, unless the number is stated with the exercise.

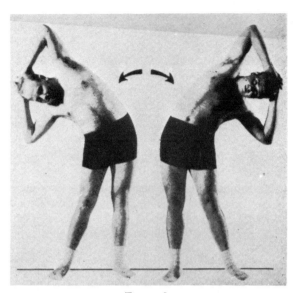

Figure 2

Running

To Develop Endurance and Speed.

1. Begin with a total distance of ½ mile and gradually increase until one mile is run each day. (Suggested routine: first slow, easy *run* for two to three minutes; then sudden, fast *sprint* for 15 to 20 yards; finally a fast *walk* for 50 yards. Repeat the sequence: run, sprint, and walk for the total distance of ½ to one mile. Practice sharp turns to each side while running.) The sprinting may be started quickly on a signal from the leader. The running should be done up and down hills; some could be done on steps or stairs, as in the stadium.

2. Run backward at best speed for 15 to 20 yards, and then quickly run forward for the same distance. Repeat two or three times.

3. Hop for 25 yards on one foot and repeat with the other foot. Hold opposite knee

high, keeping hands on hips. Repeat two
or three times.

To Condition Ankles (Figure 1).

Place chalk lines 15 inches on either side of
a center line. Run with the feet apart,
placing feet on outer lines.

Standing

To Increase Flexibility of the Trunk.

Side Bender (Figure 2).

Cadence: Moderately slow.

Starting position: Stand with feet apart,
hands clasped over head and arms straight.

Movement:

1. With the right knee straight, bend body
   sideward slowly and as far as possible
   to the right.
2. Return to starting position.
3. Repeat (1) to left.

Repeat 10 times for each side.

Trunk Twister (Figure 3).

Cadence: Moderately slow.

Starting position: Stand with feet apart,
hands behind head and knees straight.

Movement:

1. With knees straight, bend body oblique-
   ly to left and bring right elbow toward
   left thigh.
2. Return to starting position.
3. With knees straight, bend body oblique-
   ly to right and bring left elbow toward
   right thigh.
4. Return to starting position.
5. With knees straight, bend forward as
   far as possible.
6. Return to starting position.
7. With knees straight, bend backward as
   far as possible.

Repeat each movement 10 times.

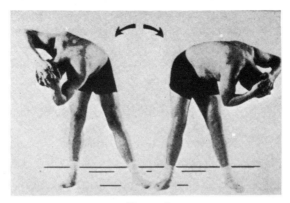

Figure 3

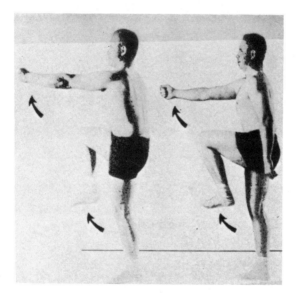

Figure 4

To Strengthen Legs and Improve Endurance.

Stationary Run (Figure 4).

Cadence: First slow, then fast, then slow.

Starting position: Stand erect, with arms at thrust and fists lightly clenched.

Movement:

1. Begin slowly and speed up somewhat, raising knees to the height of the hips.

67

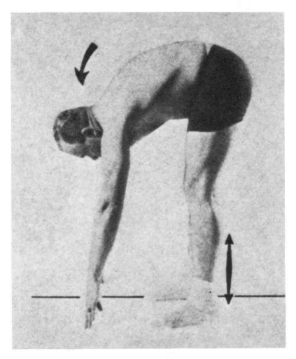

Figure 5

2. Run for a while at full speed, raising
   knees forcibly, then slow down.
   From ½ to one minute should be spent on
   this exercise.

To Stretch Hamstring Muscles.

Hamstring Stretch (Figure 5).
   Cadence: Moderate.
   Starting position: Stand erect.
   Movement:

1. Bend forward at the waist, with knees
   straight, and touch ground between
   feet.
2. Relax slightly and "bob" downward
   again, touching ground from 6 to 8
   inches farther forward.

68

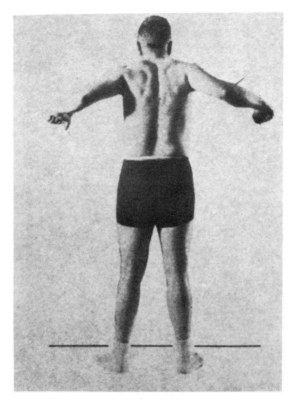

Figure 6

3. Repeat (2), touching ground still farther forward.
4. Return to starting position.

To Strengthen Upper Back Muscles and to Stretch Muscles of the Chest.

Shoulder-Blade Squeezer (Figure 6).
Cadence: Slow.
Starting position: Stand erect, with feet together and arms forward and level with shoulders.
Movement:
1. Swing arms sideward and backward as far as possible.
2. Relax slightly and swing arms backward again.

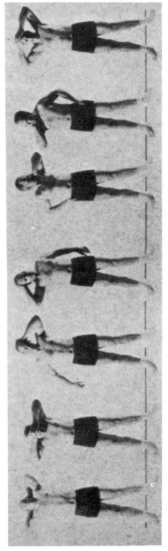

Figure 7

3. Repeat (2).
4. Return to starting position.

To Strengthen Muscles of the Neck.

Neck Firm (Figure 7).
    Cadence: Moderate-to-slow.
    Starting position: Stand erect, with fingers laced behind head.
    Movement: (isometric)

1. Keeping elbows back, raise chest high, pulling head backward against resistance of hands. Repeat five times.
2. With fingers laced and held against forehead, push head forward against resistance. Repeat five times.
3. Hold left hand against left side of head. Attempt to touch ear to left shoulder, resisting motion with left hand. Repeat five times.
4. Reverse (3) to right side. Repeat five times.
5. Rotation. Place right hand on right side of lower jaw. Attempt to turn head to the right against resistance. Repeat five times.
6. Rotation. Reverse of (5). Repeat five times.
7. Circumduction. Tense all muscles of neck and move head in complete range of movement, first in clockwise motion and then counter-clockwise. Repeat five times in each direction.

Sitting

To Strengthen Abdominal Muscles.

Abdominal Strengthening—Sit-up (Figure 8).
    Cadence: Moderate.
    Starting position: Lie on back, with knees bent and hands behind neck, feet held flat on ground by a teammate.
    Movement:

1. Come to sitting position by "curling"

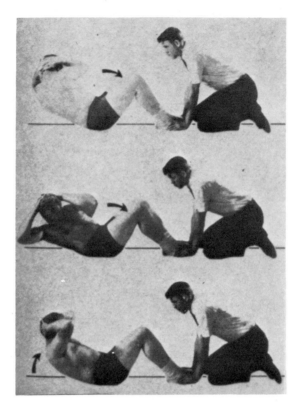

Figure 8

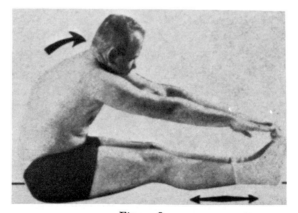

Figure 9

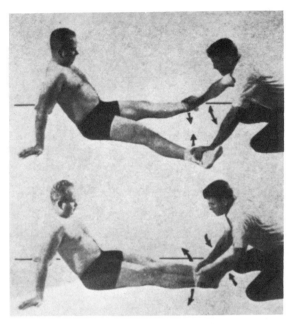

Figure 10

the trunk, touching right elbow to left knee.

2. Relax slowly to recumbent position.
3. Repeat, touching right elbow to left knee first and then left elbow to right knee.
4. Come to sitting position, bringing head to between the flexed knees.

Repeat 10 to 30 times.

To Stretch Back and Hamstrings.

Hamstring Stretch (Figure 9).
Cadence: Moderate.

Starting position: Sit with knees straight.
Movement:

1. Bend forward and touch toes or grasp ankles while pulling trunk forward as far as possible.
2. "Bounce" downward three times.
3. Return to starting position.

Repeat five to 10 times.

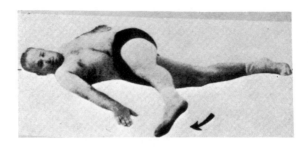

Figure 11

To Strengthen the Muscles of the Groin.

Groin Strengthening (Figure 10).
Cadence: Moderate.
Starting position: Sit with legs outstretched
and hands at side or in back of trunk for
support, legs grasped at the ankles and
held firmly by a teammate.
Movement: (isometric)
1. Move the legs against resistance of the
teammate in strong efforts to bring the
feet together.
2. Repeat above, except move legs apart
against resistance.

Lying On Back (Supine Position)

*To Increase Flexibility of the Trunk and to
Strengthen Muscles of the Upper Back.*

Leg-Back Stretch (Figure 11).
Cadence: Moderate.
Starting position: Lie flat on back, with arms
outstretched at right angles to the trunk
and palms flat on ground.
Movement:
With knees stiff and without moving
shoulders, raise one leg to perpendicular
position and swing it across the body
until foot touches opposite hand.
Repeat 10 to 15 times for each leg.

*To Strengthen the Muscles of the
Legs and Trunk.*

Bicycle (Figure 12).

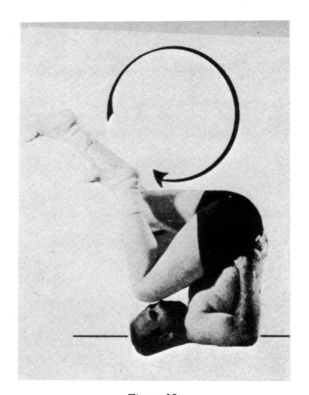

Figure 12

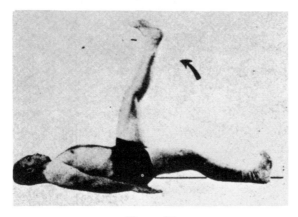

Figure 13

Cadence: Moderate.
Starting position: Support body on shoulders, with elbows on ground and hands on hips.

75

Movement:
> Raise legs and body as high as necessary in order to move feet and legs as rapidly as possible in an alternate motion, as in riding a bicycle.

Repeat 20 to 30 times.

To Strengthen Legs and Abdominal Muscles.

Leg Raiser-Straight Leg Raising (Figure 13).
Cadence: Moderate.

> Starting position: Lie on back with feet together and arms at side of body.
> Movement:
> 1. Raise left leg upward to the vertical.
> 2. With knees straight, lower left leg and at the same time raise right leg to the vertical.

Repeat 20 to 30 times.

To Strengthen the Muscles of Neck and Back.

Wrestler's Bridge (Figure 14).

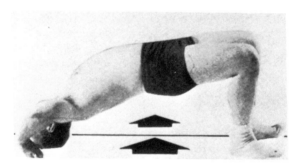

Figure 14

Cadence: Moderate-to-slow.

> Starting position: Lie on back, with feet drawn up about a foot below hips, knees bent slightly farther than a right angle, fists clenched and placed by side of head, elbows forward.
> Movement:
> 1. Raise the body as high as possible, resting the weight on fists, head, and feet.

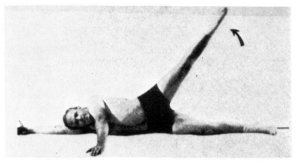

Figure 15

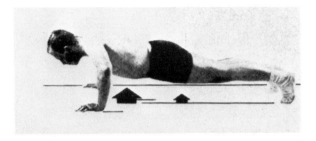

Figure 16

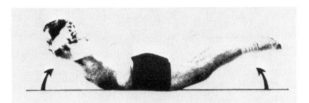

Figure 17

2. Recover to starting position.
Repeat three to five times.

To Strengthen Muscles of the Hips.

Leg-Side Raiser (Figure 15).
Cadence: Moderate.
Starting position: Lie full length on right side, with head resting on outstretched right arm.
Movement:
1. Raise left leg as high as possible, keeping knee straight and leg in line with the body.

2. Repeat on left side, raising right leg as high as possible.

Repeat 20 to 30 times on each side.

Lying On Abdomen (Prone Position)

To Strengthen Muscles of Arms.

Push-up (Figure 16).
Cadence: Moderate.
Starting position: Rest with hands on ground on either side of chest, knees and hips straight.
Movement:
1. Bend elbows and touch chest to ground, keeping body straight.
2. Straighten elbows, raising body to straight line.
Repeat 10 to 20 times.

To Strengthen Muscles of Back and Neck.

Back Strengthening (Figure 17).
Cadence: Moderate.
Starting position: Lie on stomach, with hands behind head.
Movement:
1. With knees straight, arch back, lifting feet, legs, head, and chest off ground.
2. Repeat with arms extended fully over head.
Do each exercise 10 to 20 times.

To Strengthen the Muscles of the Extremities.

All Fours (Figure 18).
Cadence: Moderate.
Starting position: Lie with weight on hands and feet.
Movement:
Walk forward, backward, and sideward on hands and feet.

To Strengthen the Muscles of the Trunk and Extremities.

Elbow Extension Press-up (Figure 19).

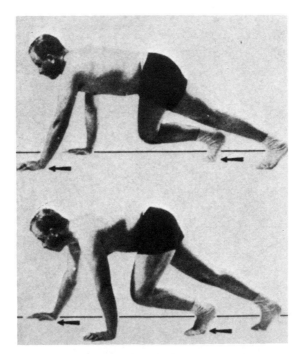

Figure 18

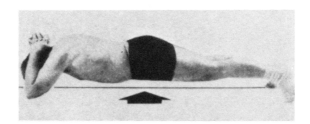

Figure 19

Cadence: Moderate.

Starting position: Lie face down with legs straight out and hands clasped behind head.

Movement:

Resting on toes and elbows, lift all other parts of the body up away from the ground. Hold for count of three.

Repeat three to five times slowly.

79

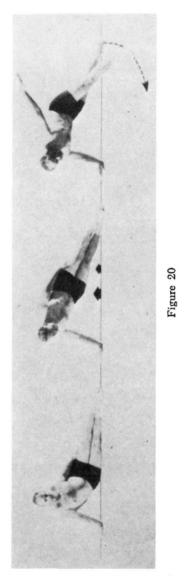

Figure 20

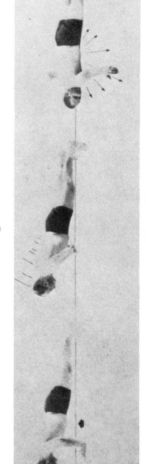

Figure 21

Hand Extension Press-up
(alternative to Elbow Extension Press-up).
  Cadence: Moderate.
  Starting position: Lie face down with legs straight out and arms straight out as far as possible above head.
  Movement:
    Keeping elbows straight, press up on toes and hands. (This can be made into a competition by seeing how long each individual can hold the position, with waistline six inches from the ground.)

To Strengthen the Muscles of the Arms and Legs.

One-Hand Spider Drill (Figure 20).
  Cadence: Moderate.
  Starting position: Sit on right thigh, with legs outstretched, trunk leaning backward and weight resting on right arm.
  Movement:
    1. Straighten body to side-leaning rest position by raising hips and thighs as high as possible.
    2. Walk in side-leaning position in a complete circle with the hand as the center of the circle of movement.
    3. Repeat (2) but use opposite hand for support and walk in side-leaning position in opposite direction.
  Repeat each exercise several times.

To Condition Chest.

Bouncer (Figure 21).
  Cadence: Moderate.
  Starting position: Lie flat on abdomen, with hands on ground.
  Movement:
    Start a push-up; quickly whip arms out to sides while dropping body to ground. Head should be back or turned to either side for the drop.
  Repeat 10 to 20 times.

References

1. Honet, J. C., Fowler, W. S., Elkins, E. C., and
   Baker, C. E.: Effects of Training and Athletic Participation on Physical Performance of High School
   Boys. Arch Phys Med 43:51, 1962.
2. Knehr, C. H., Dill, D. B., and Neufeld, W.: Training and Its Effects on Man at Rest and at Work.
   Amer J Physiol 136:148, 1942.
3. The Forty-third Annual Official Handbook. Minnesota State High School League, 375 pp, 1965-
   1966.

Medical Preparation
for the Olympic Games

Merritt H. Stiles, MD

In past Olympiads, the US Olympic Medical and Training Services Committee functioned primarily as a personnel selection and supply committee of lay members—with medical problems handled by team physicians. The prospect of having to compete at Mexico City in the XIX Olympiad introduced two major problems, that of competing at an altitude considerably higher than that of any previous summer games and the well-recognized problem of enteritis. The primary step taken by the US Olympic Committee to meet these challenges was the appointment of a broad-based Medical and Training Services Committee, after consultation with the American College of Sports Medicine, the American Medical Association Committee on the

Medical Aspects of Sports, other organizations, and numerous individuals. Because of the physiologic problems which were anticipated, an Advisory Panel on Sports Physiology was also appointed.

An early responsibility of the Medical and Training Services Committee was the selection of medical, nursing, and training personnel for the Olympic Games and for the Pan-American Games to be held in the summer of 1967. Since no salaries are paid, the Medical and Training Services Committee depends on volunteers to fill these positions. It is gratifying to report that the committee's principal problem was that of having to choose among the many highly qualified volunteers. It was decided that Daniel F. Hanley, MD, who had had previous Olympic Games experience, serve as head team physician for all quadrennial events. Otherwise, it was planned to use different physicians, nurses, and trainers at the various events, to take the greatest advantage possible of the available talent.

X Winter Olympic Games

The Medical and Training Services Committee's principal concern regarding the winter games at Grenoble, France, was the lack of authorization for sufficient medical and training personnel to care for US team members housed in five widely separated areas, some as much as 50 miles apart over narrow mountain roads. There seemed to be no possible way in which the two team physicians, one nurse, and two trainers allotted could provide adequate care for the widely scattered athletes. The French did plan to establish first-aid stations in most competition and housing areas. Such facilities could care for emergencies, but they would be of little, if any, help in settling such important questions as to whether an ailing athlete was able, or in condition, to compete in a given event.

Thanks in large part to the US Olympic Committee president, Douglas F. Roby, the International Olympic Committee and the Grenoble Organizing Committee approved the assignment of additional personnel. Trainers were stationed at Chamrousse with the Alpine team and at Autrans with the Nordic team, leaving only the relatively small Luge team without either a resident physician or trainer, since fortunately the bobsled team at Alpe d'Huez had a physician member. The outlying teams kept in close touch with the team physicians in Grenoble, the team physicians visiting the outlying groups as necessary.

The Grenoble Olympic Organizing Committee had set up well-equipped first-aid stations at each competition and housing area, staffed by physicians from the military services, or by physicians whose residency training was interrupted for the period of the games. United States team physicians were notified promptly in the event of injury of a competitor. If the injury was serious enough to require evacuation by helicopter to the general hospital at

La Tronche in suburban Grenoble, team physicians were usually able to be at the hospital by the time the injured competitor arrived. All definitive care was in the hands of US physicians.

The team housing in Grenoble and the outlying areas was excellent, the best ever in the opinion of experienced Olympic officials. Food was, if anything, too appetizing and too abundant. While an unusual number of accidents was experienced by US team members, it was possible to handle them promptly and effectively.

XIX Olympiad

Gastroenteritis.—The Medical and Training Services Committee's principal concern during the current quadrennium has been with two problems presented by the XIX Olympiad—that of gastroenteritis and that of competition at Mexico City's moderate altitude of about 7,349 feet. In considering the gastroenteritis problem, the committee noted that, in spite of the great prevalence of traveler's diarrhea, it was still not well understood. It was noted that there were many variations and degrees of severity and that prophylactic and therapeutic medication was only partially successful. It was further noted that in approximately 50% of an exposed group enteritis would develop during the first week and usually last a day or two. However, some of the affected individuals might remain ill a considerably longer period; in some, recurrent attacks might develop; and in some of the original group, the initial attacks might develop two or three weeks after the first exposure.[1-7] On the basis of these observations and with the confirmation (through a study by Nicholas and his co-workers [see page 757], financed by Olympic funds) that the prophylactic use of nonabsorbable sulfonamides would not have a deleterious effect on athletic performance, the Medical and Training Services Committee felt that the only justifiable approach was to adopt all possible preventive measures, and it made the following recommendations[8-10]:

1. Conduct allowable altitude training in the United States.
2. Instruct athletes, coaches, and others in
    (a) Importance of personal hygiene.
    (b) Risks of unsafe food and beverages.
    (c) Avoidance of raw foods and fruit.
3. Provide safe water and beverage supplies.

4. Secure best quality food available.
5. Prepare, cook, and serve food under safest conditions obtainable.
6. Enforce strictest possible hygiene for cooks and food handlers.
7. Use disposable dishes and utensils when possible.
8. Provide food and beverage for use when away from Olympic Village.

A visit to Villa Olimpica Planning Headquarters during the Tercera Competencia Deportiva Internacional (Little Olympics) in October 1967 proved reassuring. The Villa Olimpica staff understand the handicaps Mexico faces in staging the XIX Olympiad and has planned accordingly. Athletes will be housed in newly built ten-floor apartment buildings, with four apartments per floor, each apartment sleeping from 11 to 13 persons, each in a single bed. Ground floors will be given over to facilities for medicine and training and to personnel in related fields. Almost an entire apartment house will be turned over to US men's teams. Women will be housed separately.

The news on food handling was particularly encouraging. There will be five or six major cooking-dining complexes, plus an international unit open 24 hours. Each complex will consist of two dining halls, seating 240 each, and a common kitchen. One cooking-dining unit will be reserved for the US and Canadian teams (both men and women) plus other English-speaking American teams, such as those from Bermuda, Jamaica, and the Virgin Islands.

Most encouraging of all was the news that a leading Mexican hotel chain and a top-caliber US catering organization had been given responsibility for selecting, training, and supervising personnel and for procuring, preparing, and serving food.

It is planned to employ cooks native to the dominant nation in each complex. Other personnel will be selected and trained locally, with frequent inspection by Mexican Public Health Service representatives as well as by their immediate superiors. Food will be purchased in Mexico, except for the articles not readily available locally and which may be brought in as exotic items. Cooking will be in the custom of the major group in the complex.

Though the water supply of Olympic Village is of excellent quality, bottled water will be supplied for beverage purposes. Box lunches and bottled water and beverages will be supplied for athletes not able to return to Olympic Village during training or competition.

With this encouraging news, the committee looks forward to effective control of the gastrointestinal tract problem, provided athletes can be successfully indoctrinated in the importance of rigid personal hygiene and in the necessity of avoiding unsafe food and fruit—a task hopefully to be accomplished through brochures and through personal contact with recent Olympic athletes scheduled to visit the various training camps.

Altitude Training.—The surprising concern expressed over the dangers of competition at Mexico City's moderate altitude of 7,349 feet served a good purpose, in that it stimulated intensive study of the processes involved in altitude acclimatization and of the mechanisms involved in conditioning itself. The results of many of these studies were presented at the International Symposium on the Effects of Altitude on Physical Performance, held at Albuquerque, NM, in March 1966, and financed in part by Olympic funds. The proceedings of the conference,[11] recommendations from the Olympic Advisory Panel on Sports Physiology, discussions with physiologists and coaches experienced in high-altitude competition, and numerous observations made in recent studies, some still unpublished, have been important in developing the opinions expressed below.

It has been estimated that over 60 million persons[11] live at altitudes of 7,000 feet or higher. This observation alone should indicate that there is no danger to life from such altitudes and that there is little difficulty in acclimatization. This conclusion is affirmed by Van Nelson's performance during the Tercera Competencia, when, with no prior altitude training, he arrived in Mexico City at midnight on Sunday and ran in the 10,000 meter race the following noon, with creditable time, though about two minutes slower than at sea level. He had no untoward symptoms, he was in superb condition when he arrived, and he had had adequate instruction in pacing.

From the standpoint of athletic performance, the only important factor is that the partial pressure of oxygen is lower than at sea level. This lower oxygen pressure is of no consequence to a healthy individual doing ordinary activities, which require only a small percentage of the available oxygen supply. The symptoms which so commonly occur in persons newly arrived at high altitude are psychological in origin, with subconscious hyperventilation[11] (reported recently in *Athletic J* 46:20 [Nov] 1965) and secondary alkalosis. In athletic competition the lower partial pressure of oxygen will have no effect on field events, nor on running or swimming events not requiring more than two minutes of maximum effort. Oxygen debt, or anaerobic capacity, which has been estimated to amount to as much as 5 to 6 liters in well-conditioned athletes,[12] is the principal factor in short-duration events, and it would not be surprising if new records were set, in view of the lowered barometric pressure.

In prolonged events, for example of 20 minutes' duration, performance is dependent largely on inspired oxygen, since, when spread out over the 20-minute period, the oxygen debt capacity of 5 to 6 liters does not amount to a great deal. (Bengt Saltin, MD, has estimated 10% at 5,000 meters and 5% at 10,000 meters.[11]) Because of the lower partial pressure of oxygen one might expect performance times to be as much as 15% to 20% slower; actually, they are usually only prolonged by 7% to 10%, because of the numerous adaptive factors. In middle-distance events, requiring ten minutes for example, the oxygen debt capacity does not need to be spread so thin, and performance times are only about 5% longer than at sea level. In events requiring only around four minutes of maximum effort, performance times are prolonged only by 3% to 4%.

The events affected will be running, swimming, cycling, rowing, or paddling events of over two minutes' duration. Team events which require interrupted effort, such as soccer-football, water polo, basketball,[11] and field hockey; and bout events, in which exertion is on a stop-and-go basis, should be little affected, since the overall effort may not require more than 75% of the available oxygen supply.

While experience has shown that adaptation to altitude does occur, the factors involved are not completely understood. Increased pulmonary ventilation is always a factor,[11] perhaps too prompt a factor in some individuals. Most, but not all, studies have shown improvement in the maximum oxygen uptake over a 10- to 14-day period[11] (A. C. DeGraff, Jr., et al, unpublished data), though not beyond this point. It has long been known that the hemoglobin level is significantly increased at higher elevations. While again not all studies made at moderate altitudes are in agreement, most have shown an early hemoconcentration with a later increase in hemoglobin level and erythrocyte count.[11] Reports of other studies have indicated that myoglobin levels may be increased,[11] that increased tissue vascularization may develop,[11] that cardiac output may increase,[11] and that the arteriovenous oxygen difference may be widened.[11] These factors combine to provide the increased oxygen delivery capacity, or maximum oxygen uptake. Available evidence also indicates that increased anaerobic capacity may be a factor in altitude adaptation.[11,13]

Though reassurance as to the absence of harmful effects may at times be a factor in improved athletic performance, experience in pacing is in all probability a more important factor. In effect, the 2-miler needs to learn to pace himself as though he were running $2\frac{1}{2}$ to 3 miles at sea level. Concern has been expressed that the slower pace might result in some degree of muscle detraining, but if so, increased "spurt" training could be corrective.[11]

Not all athletes adapt equally well to altitude. This may be due to psychological factors in some. In others it may be due to lessened pulmonary diffusion of oxygen, though this can be overcome to some extent by increased ventilation. Though some studies have shown minor improvement at moderate altitude over a longer period, most adaptive changes apparently occur within a two- to three-week period. There seems to be general agreement that adaptation is fastest in the athlete who is in good condition when he arrives at altitude,[11] who trains vigorously,[11] and who runs time trials during his first day or two.[13] The old myth, "Take it easy the first few days at altitude," seems to be well exploded as far as moderate altitudes are concerned. In fact, there is evidence that "taking it easy" for a few days may result in a significant degree of detraining.[11] This is readily understood when one considers the factor which Favour has stressed,[11] the marked degree of cross-adaptation between altitude acclimatization and a vigorous conditioning program at any altitude, a degree of cross-adaptation so great as to suggest that both are essentially the same process, the principal difference being one of degree. Both produce a relative hypoxemia, followed in turn by increased pulmonary ventilation, increased cardiac output, an increase in respiratory pigments, increased tissue vascularization, and widened arteriovenous oxygen difference, all of which combine to increase maximum oxygen uptake and delivery. There is evidence also that anaerobic capacity increases in both situations.

Recovery times should be about the same at moderate altitude as at sea level[11]; some experienced coaches even feel altitude recovery time may be shorter[14] (*Athletic J* 46:20 [Nov] 1965). Recovery from short-duration events consists largely of repaying the oxygen debt. The "alactate" portion, approximately one half the total, is half repaid in about 30 seconds at sea level.[12] Since ventilation is close to capacity during this period, repayment of this portion of the debt might take 35 to 40 seconds at moderate altitude. Repayment of the remaining portion of the alactate debt, which takes about three minutes at sea level, and repayment of the "lactate" portion of the debt, a much more gradual process, should take no longer at moderate altitude, since ventilation is at a much lower level. Recovery from prolonged endurance events, where muscle fatigue and glycogen depletion become important factors, will take longer, although the time should not be significantly greater than at sea level.

A number of reports by competent investigators have indicated that performance may be improved by alternating periods of high-altitude and low-altitude training[13] (J. T. Daniels, unpublished data), though other studies have not confirmed this observation. Still other studies have indicated that performance at altitude may be improved by altitude training the previous year (B. Saltin, personal communication, Oct 1967). The reasons for such improvement are not clear, unless altitude variations stress adaptive mechanisms to a greater degree than does training at a single altitude. While confirmation of these observations will depend on repeated studies, it seems abundantly clear that no harmful effects are associated with repeated episodes of altitude training or with interruption of a period of training at high altitude by a return to a lower altitude.

On the basis of the observations and opinions cited, the following recommendations were made to the games planning committee and to the individual sports committees:

1. No danger exists in altitude competition itself.
2. Most symptoms at moderate altitude are psychological, from hyperventilation.
3. New records are possible in field and short-duration events.
4. Performance times will be prolonged in middle- and long-distance events.
5. Acclimatization and improved performance at altitude result from the following:
   A. Cross-adaptation with conditioning programs.
      (1) Improvement in maximum oxygen uptake.
         (a) Increased pulmonary ventilation.
         (b) Increased cardiac output.
         (c) Increase in respiratory pigments.
         (d) Increased tissue vascularization.
         (e) Widened arteriovenous oxygen difference.
      (2) Increased anaerobic capacity.
   B. Reassurance.
   C. Experience in pacing.
6. Altitude acclimatization is fastest:
   A. In well-conditioned athletes.
   B. With vigorous training.
   C. With early time trials.
7. Recovery times are essentially the same as at sea level.
8. The maximum allowable training should be conducted at altitude for competitors in events requiring more than two minutes of maximum effort.
9. Shorter periods of altitude training are suitable for other competitors.
10. Repeated periods of altitude training may improve performance.

References

1. Thomas, C.L.: Gastroenteritis of Travelers in Athletes, presented at Postgraduate Course on Sports Medicine, American Academy of Orthopedic Surgeons, Oklahoma City, Aug 15, 1967.
2. Gordon, J.E.: Acute Diarrheal Diseases, *Amer J Med Sci* 248:345-365 (Sept) 1965.
3. Kean, B.H., and Tucker, H.A.: *The Traveler's Medical Guide for Physicians,* Springfield, Ill: Charles C Thomas, Publisher, 1966.
4. Kean, B.H.: The Diarrhea of Travelers to Mexico: Summary of Five Year Study, *Ann Intern Med* 59:605-614 (Nov) 1963.
5. Hardy, A.V.: Current Problems in the Enteric Infections, *Med Clin N Amer* 51:609-615 (May) 1967.
6. Dubos, R.J., et al: The Indigenous Flora of the Intestinal Tract, *Dis Colon Rectum* 10:23-24 (Jan) 1967.
7. Philbrook, F.R., and Gordon, J.E.: "Diarrhea and Dysentery," in *Preventive Medicine in W.W. II,* Office of the Surgeon General, Department of the Army, 1958, vol 4.
8. Kean, B.H., et al: The Diarrhea of Travelers: V. Prophylaxis With Phthalylsulfathiazole and Neomycin Sulfate, *JAMA* 180:367-371 (May 5) 1962.
9. Giffin, R.B., and Gaines, S.: Diarrhea in a US Battle Group in Thailand, *Milit Med* 129:546-550 (June) 1964.
10. Gordon, J.E. (ed.): *Control of Communicable Disease in*

Man, ed 10, New York: American Public Health Association, 1965, p 83.

11. Goddard, R. (ed.): *Proceedings of the International Symposium on the Effects of Altitude on Physical Performance,* Chicago: Athletic Institute, 1967.

12. Dill, D.B., and Sacktor, B.: Exercise and the Oxygen Debt, *J Sport Med* 2:66-72 (June) 1962.

13. Balke, B.: Effects of Training at Sea Level and at Altitude, presented in Symposium on Exercise and Altitude, Milano, 1966.

14. Arnesen, A.V.: The Comparison in Cross Country Between Altitude and Sea Level Races, *USTCA Quart Rev,* June 1966.

Injury Prevention
in Skiing and Snowmobiling

MERRITT H. STILES, M.D.

While skiing and snowmobiling are similar in being winter sports dependent on snow cover, they differ widely from the standpoint of accident potential and injury prevention. Terrain-equipment-human relationship is simple in skiing, essentially that between an individual and snow-covered terrain, somewhat complicated by the interposition of a pair of slippery boards. In snowmobiling the direct relation between individual and snow is minor, unless he is stranded by equipment breakdown in a wilderness. The relationship between snowmobile and snow-covered terrain is more important, though still less important than the relationship between man and machine. The risks of accident and injury are similar to those that exist whenever a human being — all too often inexperienced, incompetent, careless or befuddled — exercises control over a powered vehicle.

ACCIDENT AND INJURY IN SKIING

In considering skiing, it is important to make a distinction between accident and injury. There are many circumstances that result in accidental falls: snow conditions, terrain conditions, the skier's maneuvers — almost all the result of interaction between skier and terrain. Yet only a very small percentage of these accidents result in significant injury, providing, of course, injury to one's pride is discounted.

terrain

Skiing is easiest on a smooth, gentle slope, although such a slope is not as safe as it might seem. *Deep snow,* heavy and wet; *hard-packed snow,* and *breakable crust* over soft snow are frequent causes of severe falls, and most skiers avoid such conditions assiduously. Steep slopes are often covered with *moguls* (rounded mounds), a hazard in themselves, but also a help in turning for the experienced skier. When a steep slope becomes hard-packed or icy it introduces the risk of a prolonged, and sometimes dangerous, slide to the bottom of the slope should the skier fall. In other snow conditions a steep slope may present the risk of avalanching. All of these hazards are greatly increased by *fog or flat light,* causing surface details to disappear. A large number of skiers, particularly beginners, concentrated in a small area, introduces another hazard: *collision* with another skier.

ability

More important than snow and terrain, however, is the ability of the skier himself. Once past the basic instruction phase many children quickly become competent by mimicking good skiers, but most older persons progress only slowly. The difficulties are compounded, of course, if the beginning skier is not in good physical condition. A study of leg fractures in 1967-68 showed that the skier himself was the principle contributing factor in more than 75 percent of the accidents.[1]

types of injury

Types of injuries observed by Garrick are listed in Table 1. It was noted that the incidence of injury was higher in young skiers and lower in adults, with a slight rise in skiers over 50. Beginning skiers had a higher incidence of injury, the incidence declining as ability improved. Female skiers had significantly more injuries than did males.[2]

TABLE 1

SKI INJURY CLASSIFICATION

Type of Injury	% of Total
Abrasions	2
Contusions	5
Lacerations	10
Musculo-tendinous	5
Ligamentous	39
Dislocations	3
Fractures	36
	100

rules of the slope

In 1963, the major national organizations involved in skiing formed the National Ski Study Group, a non-policy-making, non-dues-paying group composed of the heads of the member organizations.* One of the study group's first activities was the formulation and promotion of Rules of the Slope, a skier's courtesy code (see box). Federation Internationale de Ski (FIS), governing body for the sport of skiing, has developed a similar code, though stressing more strongly a skier's obligation to help others in distress. The study group encouraged lift safety codes, now in effect in most states with ski areas, and worked closely with the National Ski Areas Association (NSAA) in establishing an international uniform trail classification and marking system, indicating relative trail difficulty.

area operators

Individual ski area operators play a major role in promoting safety through slope maintenance, in grooming to remove rocks, brush piles and other obstacles; in packing deep snow so it can be negotiated more easily by the average skier; in cutting down moguls; and breaking up and dragging runs that have become too hard-packed or icy.

---

*NATIONAL SKI STUDY GROUP

National Ski Areas Association
National Ski Patrol System
Professional Ski Instructors of
    America
Ski Industries America
United States Forest Service
United States Ski Association
United States Ski Writers
    Association

Advisory member: National Safety
    Council

Added members: Ski Specialists
    Guild; Ski Retailers International

Standing committee: National Com-
    mittee on Skiing Safety

instruction

Since skiing is a learned technique, instruction is a major safety factor. Beginning skiers of mature years require patient and prolonged instruction, with periodic brushing up even after they are relatively experienced. The Professional Ski Instructors of America has developed standard teaching techniques and student classification methods so that a skier may move from one school to another around the country with minimum adjustment.

clothing

Warm, comfortable clothing is important, to prevent chilling without impairing free movement. Modern skis are in general shorter, lighter, more flexible, with a smoother running surface, and consequently more easily handled. Boots are higher and stiffer, providing better edge control but also introducing the complication of boot-top rather than ankle fractures. The most important equipment item in injury prevention is the binding which fastens the ski to the boot. Modern releasable bindings, properly adjusted, will usually release the boot from the ski in a high-speed fall, particularly on a steep slope. A fall on a gentler slope, at slower speed, may not produce the force needed to release the boot if the ski tip becomes buried, and the resultant slow, twisting fall may result in injury. Moreover, even the best binding may be of little value unless it is properly adjusted.[3,4]

physical condition

Excellent physical condition is an important factor in safety as well as in the enjoyment of skiing. Preferably this should be on a year-around basis, and not just preseason. And what might be called "mental condi-

PREVENTION OF INJURY

RULES OF THE SLOPE
A Skiers Courtesy Code

1. All skiers shall ski under control, in such a manner that a skier can avoid other skiers or objects.

2. An overtaking skier shall avoid the skier below him.

3. Skiers approaching each other on opposite traverses shall pass to the right.

4. Skiers shall not stop in a location which will obstruct a trail, not be visible from above, or impede progress of other skiers.

5. A skier entering a trail or slope from a side or intersecting trail shall first check for approaching skiers.

6. A standing skier shall check for approaching downhill skiers before starting.

7. When walking or climbing in a ski area, skis should be worn, and the walker or climber shall keep to the side of the slope.

8. All skiers shall wear straps or other devices to prevent runaway skis.

9. Skiers shall keep off closed trails and posted areas and shall observe all traffic signs and other regulations as prescribed by the ski area.

---

tioning" is important: education in the hazards of various snow and terrain conditions, and good judgment in the selection of runs and slopes to be skied under prevailing circumstances. Measures to lessen risk of ski injury are: slope grooming and maintenance; lift maintenance; trail and closed area marking; use of dependable equipment, including releasable bindings; knowledge of binding adjustment methods; adequate instruction and practice; education in ski rules of the slope, and good physical condition.

binding adjustment service

Efforts to lessen injury have actually produced favorable results as reported by O'Malley, Table 2. Mount Tom Ski Area, Holyoke, Massachusetts, has provided checking and adjustment service of bindings, without cost, to 25,000 skiers.[5]

grooming the slopes

When asked why Vail was packing out so many more runs and slopes than it had in earlier years, Robert Parker, Vail's Marketing Manager, stated, "We feel it is an important safety measure; our injury rate is down from 3.72 per 1,000 ski man days to 2.6," though Garrick[2] was of the opinion that the most important contributing factor, accounting for about half of the improvement, was the improved proficiency of the average skier.

Mr. Paul Copello has stated, "Actually, the most dangerous part of the skier's day is the drive home. Looking at claims paid over the years it becomes apparent that skiers, tired from a day on slopes or in the lodge, are apt to get involved in traffic accidents." Mr. Copello adds, "Walking around frozen streets in ski boots is potentially more dangerous than skiing itself. Wear something

TABLE 2

COMPARATIVE INJURY STATISTICS

Mt. Tom Ski Area, Holyoke, Massachusetts

Years	Man Days Skiing	Injuries No.	Rate per 1,000 M.D.S.	Fractures No.	Rate per 1,000 M.D.S.
1960-65	438,022	2,126	4.85	324	0.74
1966-67	120,613	489	4.05	83	0.68
1967-68	102,940	368	3.58	68	0.66

more appropriate."[6]

While ski areas have on occasion had sewage disposal and comparable problems, and while timber cutting for runs and lifts was all too often done in conspicuous and unattractive straight lines in the past, and not with an overall landscaping plan as at present, the terrain involved has been relatively small, and any resultant harm limited.

ACCIDENT AND INJURY IN SNOWMOBILING

The snowmobile has demonstrated its non-sport usefulness in many ways: in allowing telephone linemen to make otherwise almost impossible wintertime repairs; in feeding snowbound stock, and in winter rescue operations where its load-carrying potential is of special value. To my knowledge there have been no significant injuries reported as a result of such use. The snowmobile injury problem arises rather from its "alluring but alarming" recreational use, driven by persons of all ages, with all degrees of experience, and by many with all too little knowledge of the whims and vagaries of self-propelled vehicles.[7]

Available reports present an alarming picture, with tragic deaths of persons of all ages.[8] Mr. John Marsh, Safety Coordinator for the Maine Department of Inland Fisheries and Game, has stated, "I put about 200,000 hunters into the woods a year and have only 50 accidents. Last season there were about 20,000 snowmobiles registered and there were more than 300 accidents.[9]

Professor Richard W. McLay of the University of Vermont surveyed 63 snowmobile accidents reported to six northern and central Vermont hospitals during the 1968-69 season.[10] Accident categories and special hazards felt to be contributing factors are listed in Table 3. Types of injuries and fracture locations are shown in Table 4. The high incidence of fractures of the spine, usually the result of jumping, is of particular interest.

97

TABLE 3

SNOWMOBILE ACCIDENT CATEGORIES AND HAZARDS

Accident categories	Number
Collision with another vehicle or object	9
Struck by snowmobile	4
Thrown due to maneuvers	13
Injured in jump	11
Injured by barbed wire or chain	7
Minor injuries	19

Special hazards	
Lack of experience	Speed
Equipment not in repair	Thin ice
Climbing over banks	Jumps
Poor visibility	Alcohol
Barbed wire	

TABLE 4

SNOWMOBILE INJURIES

Type	Number
Fractures and dislocations	67
Sprains	14
Lacerations	12
Contusions	8
Foreign body	1
Fatality	1
	103

Fracture locations	Number
Skull and face	4
Clavicle, scapula, ribs, sternum	9
Arm	11
Spine	15
Pelvis	2
Leg	27

SNOWMOBILE DON'TS

Don't drive on highway.

Don't drive on railroad right-of-way.

Don't tailgate.

Don't cut across another's right-of-way.

Don't go on ice without knowing thickness.

Don't jump a snowbank without knowing what is on other side.

Don't be a show-off.

Don't let children operate snowmobile alone.

Don't put hands or feet near track while driving.

Don't travel unfrequented areas alone.

Don't panic.

SNOWMOBILE DO'S

Do obtain operating instructions.

Do learn to know your machine.

Do keep it in good repair.

Do make sure snowmobile is secure when on its trailer.

Do come to a full stop before crossing highway.

Do put one knee on seat for bumpy terrain or sidehill.

Do leave alcohol alone before and when operating snowmobile.

Do go more slowly if children are aboard.

Do lengthen throttle cable for children's use.

Do use towbar if pulling trailer.

Do have adequate light for nighttime driving.

Do follow marked trails at night.

Do travel with extra caution in unknown areas.

Do carry emergency supplies on safari.

prevention

The National Safety Council has taken the lead in promoting safety in snowmobiling. Besides gathering records to permit the identification of risk factors, it has published safety education data, recommended regulatory procedures and, in cooperation with a leading manufacturer, has developed and promoted safety booklets, listing both "Don'ts" and "Do's." (See above.) Legislation is required, including where not now in effect, registration and licensing of equipment, licensing of operators with age limitations, restrictions on horsepower for recreational vehicles, headlight standards, tail-light requirements, and regulations on highway use.

Cooperation of volunteer and trade organizations with the National Safety Council in educational and regulatory programs, and in such safety programs as trail marking, would materially brighten snowmobiling's future.

There are some encouraging developments in snowmobiling. Professor McLay reported that one snowmobile club in Vermont, with about 85 members, had only one major injury during the winter of 1968-69, a broken leg, suggesting that participating in a club dedicated to courtesy and safety might make a snowmobiler less accident-prone.[11]

Snowmobiles range widely, however, and disturbing observations have been reported. A winter kill of fish in Coon Lake, Wisconsin, was traced to a reduction of dissolved oxygen in the water. Heavy snowmobile use had compacted the snow over the ice, making it opaque and restricting the amount of sunlight getting to aquatic plants which need it for photosynthesis and for the production of oxygen.[12]

Hunting coyotes by snowmobile was so effective in Ontario that the price of a coyote pelt fell from $25.00 to $5.00. But there were unexpected side effects. Mice and other rodents, ordinarily kept under control by coyotes, proliferated and destroyed field crops to a serious extent. Snowmobiles have also been reported as doing serious direct damage to winter wheat, when operated in fields with insufficient snow cover.

The damaging effects of the noisy, ubiquitous snowmobile in driving wild life away from its usual winter haunts, and in destroying the winter quiet on which wild life depends for self-renewal, can only be guessed at.[9] Nor is the snowmobile the end of the environment-altering line. Already in production are all-terrain-vehicles (ATV's) capable of traveling on sand and marsh as well as on snow, and even capable of traveling over logs. Also in production is the S P D Tricat, and the Air Gator, a snowboat powered by an aircraft type engine. Of even greater concern are the one-seat, eight-foot Hoverhornet, expected to sell for less than a thousand dollars, and the fifteen-foot Hoverhawk, hovercraft whose horrendous roars may make the typical snowmobile whine sound like a gentle zephyr.[13]

REFERENCES

1 Garis, R., Reducing ski injuries, presented before Winter Sports Safety Congress, Chicago, Illinois, October 28, 1969.

2 Garrick, J. G., The epidemiology of ski injuries, presented before American College of Sports Medicine, Albuquerque, New Mexico, May 9, 1970.

3 Lipe, G. C., Factual evidence of errors and omissions which produce release binding malfunction, presented before Northwestern Medical Association, Sun Valley, Idaho, February 10, 1970.

4 Outwater, J. O. and Ettlinger, C. F., An engineer looks at ski bindings, presented before Winter Sports Safety Congress, Chicago, Illinois, October 28, 1969.

5 O'Malley, R. D., A ski area's approach to safety, presented before Northeastern Medical Association, Vail, Colorado, March 2, 1970.

6 Copello, P., How safe is skiing? Western Ski Time 3: 16-17 (December 25) 1968.

7 Editorial, The alluring but alarming snowmobile, Family Safety 28:4-7 (Winter) 1969.

8 Fleming, J. P., Safety, presented before International Snowmobile Conference, Albany, N. Y., May 20, 1969.

9 Olsen, J., Bad show out in the cold snow, Sports Illustrated 32:28-35 (March 16) 1970.

10 McLay, R. E. and Chism, S. E., A snowmobile accident study, presented before International Snowmobile Conference, Albany, N. Y., May 20-21, 1969.

11 Chism, S. E. and Soule, A. B., Snowmobile injuries, JAMA 209:1672-1674 (September 15) 1969.

12 Editorial, Snowmobiles a menace to fish, Environmental Action Bulletin 8:6 (May 9) 1970.

13 Environmental Brief, Here comes another unnecessary danger to wildlife, Environmental Action Bulletin 8:1 (May 30) 1970.

Orthopedic Aspects and Safety Factors in Snow Skiing

MARK R. HARWOOD, M.D.

GERALD L. STRANGE, M.D.

SKIING IS POPULAR despite a high incidence of injury as witness this poetic warning written by Stephen Leech, our local executive secretary, from the December, 1964, *Onondaga County Medical Bulletin.*

T'is the Season

Away golf clubs and away outboards
　　Here come the roaring, thundering hordes
Of skiers who, though properly shod
　　Often wind up at the orthopod.

So skiers stock up with crutches and braces
　　'Ere starting off to the slalom races
For just ahead of every Christy turn
　　Stands the orthopod with a living to earn.

So tighten your laces and check your ski poles
　　While golfers lament and turn into moles
But just be careful before the season is done
　　Or only the orthopod will have won.

There are almost 2 million skiers, and this number is growing fast. *The New York Times* estimated that there will be

Presented at the 159th Annual Meeting of the Medical Society of the State of New York, New York City, Section on Orthopedic Surgery, February 18, 1965.

$75 million spent on ski equipment and clothing this year.

The incidence of injury according to the various reports averages approximately 0.7 per cent, meaning that for each thousand people skiing in one day there will be about 7 injured.

Preparations for skiing

For those who do not ski, it might be well to go over the material needed for skiing. It is. important to be warmly dressed to prevent frostbite. The top of the hill may be much colder than the bottom, particularly with the wind blowing. For each mph of wind velocity, the temperature is decreased 1 F. The use of net under clothing provides a layer of warm air next to the body, and long duofold underwear should protect against extreme weather. Thermal socks over a pair of silk socks and boots that are not laced too tightly over the toes will prevent the toes from freezing. The boots require lateral support and a precise fit, especially for present style short swing turns. A desirable boot is one that makes skier and skis a single unit without sacrificing the skier's comfort. A firm boot, moderately high with a cushioned inner boot, provides a good support for the ankle and cuts down on the incidence of ankle fracture. With a really stiff boot high up the leg, the effect of the shearing pin mechanism of a malleolus fracture in external rotation strain is lost and all the force is transmitted to the tibia and knee.[1] Poles are necessary for support in climbing and for making proper unweighted turns. They are made with sharp points and when waving in the air can produce injury. This is one cause for the increase in eye injuries. Skis can be made of wood, plastic, or aluminum and have a steel offset edge. Lacerations from these edges are not uncommon, and some will require many sutures.

TABLE I. Sprague's table of speeds attained by a
190-pound skier under optimum conditions[9]

Slope Angle (Degrees)	Velocity (Mph)
3	24
5	34
10	52
20	75
30	92
45	110

Causes of accidents

Causes of accidents on the ski slopes are varied, but more than half of them occur because the skiers are out of control. You can see why if you study the speeds attained with specific degrees of slope (Table I).[2]

A 150-pound skier at 30 mph has a 6,600 feet per second momentum. This would generate a force of 15 g if he stopped within 2 feet (Fig. 1).[3] If you attach a 6-foot ski to a foot-long appendage of rigid design, a torque of a 3-foot lever arm is added to the forces mentioned. This torsional force, mostly in external rotation, is a dynamic factor both in fracture and soft-tissue damage which we have tried to study (Table II).

Looking over the statistics of the past five years in the local areas within 25 miles of Syracuse, where we have five major ski areas, and including those injuries which came into our office after first being seen or treated in another area, we studied 854 and verified 650 cases and list the following probable torsional strain injuries accounting for 64 per cent or 417 of the total. In comparing these with the statistics of leading articles of recent years, we note the gradual increase in knee and tibia injuries (Table III).

A simple fracture of the lateral malleolus used to be the most common injury and was therefore called a "ski fracture" (Fig. 2A). There may be associated subluxation with tear of the deltoid as demonstrated by a stress film (Fig. 2B).

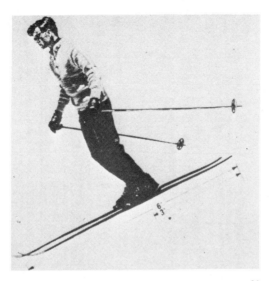

FIGURE 1. Momentum of 150-pound skier at 30 mph is 6,600 feet per second, generating force of 15 g if stopping at 2 feet.[3]

TABLE II. Total injuries 1960 to 1964

Type of Injury	Number	Per Cent
Fractures of shaft of tibia and tibia or fibula	105	16
Fractures of foot and ankle	55	8
Other fractures; upper extremity, spine	30	5
Shoulder dislocations	9	1
Sprains of knee	142	22
Sprains of ankle	115	18
Other sprains and contusions	54	8
Lacerations	140	21
TOTAL	650	

The tearing of the anterior, inferior, tibio-fibular ligament may be produced by the same external rotation force as the initial injury. If the force continues upward, a fracture of the fibula at higher levels may occur (Fig. 3A). If the torsional force is sudden, the tibial insertion of the tibio-

105

TABLE III. Increase in knee and tibia injuries

Type of Injury	Sun Valley, Idaho, 1960 to 1961[6]		Mt. Snow, Vermont, 1960 to 1961[2]		Laurentians, Canada, ? to 1964[7]	Syracuse, New York, 1960 to 1964	
	Number	Per Cent	Number	Per Cent	Per Cent	Number	Per Cent
Sprain of foot or ankle	402	27	147	21	19	115	18
Sprain of knee	235	16	113	16	20	142	22
Fracture of foot or ankle	152	10	120	18	24	55	8
Fracture of shaft, tibia, or fibula	83	5	90	13	16	105	16
TOTALS	872	58	470	68	79	417	64

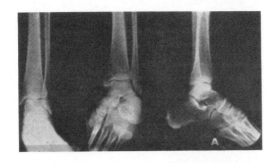

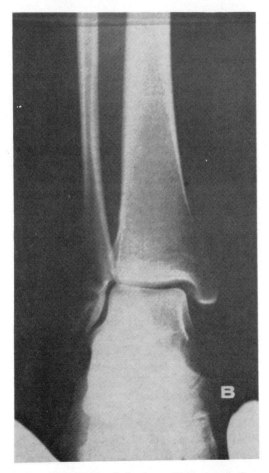

FIGURE 2. (A) Simple fracture of lateral malleolus.
(B) Associated subluxation with tear of deltoid.

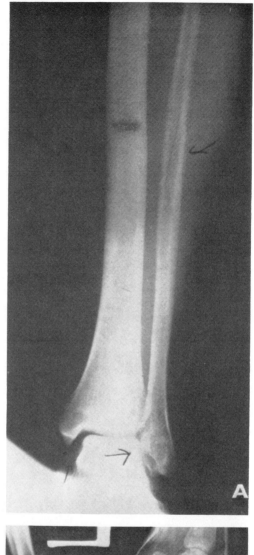

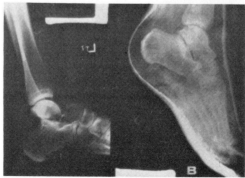

FIGURE 3. (A) Fracture of fibula at higher level. (B) Fracture of neck of talus.

fibular ligament is avulsed, and a diastasis of the ankle joint occurs.

If the boots do not fit or are too loose, the torsion effect may produce both foot

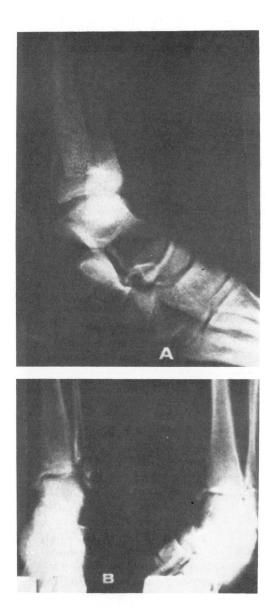

FIGURE 4. (A) Fracture of anterior portion of os calcis and subtalar dislocation. (B) Bimalleolar fracture, dislocation of ankle.

and ankle injuries. A twenty-five-year-old secretary borrowed boots, fell in the soft snow, and dislocated her subtalar joint fracturing the neck of the talus (Fig. 3B).

One of our anesthetists had new boots and wanted to take one more run even though his boots hurt him; he loosened up the lacings and, on this last run, took a spill which produced a bimalleolar fracture dislocation of the ankle, fracture of the anterior portion of the os calcis, and a subtalar dislocation (Fig. 4). Now, a year later, he limps and has mild discomfort at the end of the day. He has no subastragalar motion but has been playing golf and skiing.

Another expert skier was just standing on a mogul when he slipped backwards pushing his foot up into severe dorsiflexion, producing an unusual fracture of the lateral process of the talus (Fig. 5A). Discussing this particular fracture in the *Journal of Bone and Joint Surgery*, Dimond[4] presented 3 cases, one of which was in a professional skier. There are only 12 cases reported in the literature, and we have also seen 3 cases recently and feel as he does that this is an intra-articular fracture which must have reduction and fixation to unite.

Knee sprains are very common, particularly in beginner skiers, and we have noted a marked increase in this injury. One of the authors has seen twenty-two knee sprains from skiing in the past two years. These all involved the medial collateral ligament and ranged from mild sprains to 2 cases with O'Donoghue triad. Two other also had medial meniscus injury. In addition, 5 of this group had associated ankle sprain, although it would seem logical that when the foot and ankle are supported by well-fitting boots with inner lacings and the torsional force is applied slowly, the transmission of this force should bypass the ankle and be applied to the medial collateral ligament in any external rotation injury.

As you would expect, spiral fracture of the tibia is common and is also increasing in frequency. In a youngster, the fibula is usually intact and of course heals readily (Fig. 5B). In an adult, the same fracture may be obtained without fracture of the fibula and will be stable although oblique (Fig. 6A). There may be the usual unstable spiral fracture with fracture of the fibula, and this may require internal fixation (Fig. 6B). About half of the tibial fractures in adults, and a smaller proportion in·youngsters are of the comminuted spiral type. Figure 7A shows the comminuted spiral fracture of a thirty-five-year-old housewife, that took six months to heal. She is not ready to ski this winter.

The force of torsion plays a minor role in the production of injuries associated with forward thrust. The skiing of moguls, jumping them, and people skiing many types of slopes where the ski point may be trapped in a downhill run throwing them forward can result in boot-top fractures of tibia and fibula (Figs. 7B and 8). In older individuals there have been several Achilles tendon ruptures from the same force.

Prevention

As noted by others,[5] there is an increased incidence of injury in the younger-age groups and a decrease in the number of accidents as skiers gain experience and beginners receive better instruction (Tables IV and V). We would like to stress some factors in prevention of injuries: (1) Reduce over-confidence, (2) have proper conditioning, (3) ski under control with courtesy, and (4) use properly adjusted release bindings.

In most areas more than 90 per cent of the skiers have some mode of release bindings, but less than half are properly adjusted to release on a slow fall.

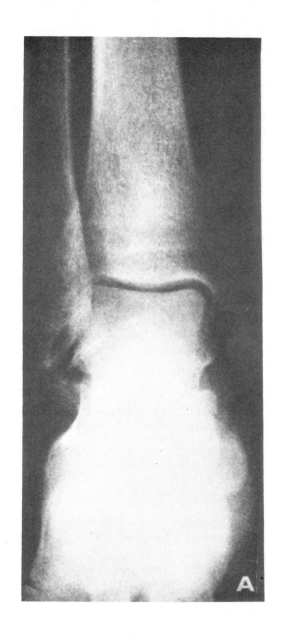

FIGURE 5. (A) Fracture of lateral process of talus.

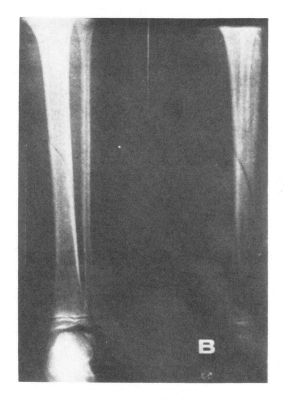

(B) Intact fibula healing readily.

The toe mechanism protects the skier from the rotational forces. Forward thrust forces are dependent on the heel release. There are over 55 types of bindings, but fewer than 12 of them are satisfactory.

Gordon Lipe[3] of Syracuse developed a testing mechanism which exerts pressure against the side of the boot, slowly building up tension until a toe release is effected (Fig. 9A). The amount of force necessary to produce this release is then measured. Mr. Lipe measured this force under varying conditions of weight and skiing ability and evolved a chart which gives a numerical setting according to the demand of the skier (Table VI). The importance of testing is evident from the fact that he has been able to tighten or loosen bindings on expert skiers as much as 100 per cent one way or the other without their being aware of the exact change he had made.

This "release check" as it is called is now in production after several years' trial. It has been made available to ski centers and ski shops who have promised to put all of their work on IBM cards and keep track of any of the injuries that occur in cases where bindings have been properly installed and properly adjusted. Perhaps these records will provide a means of determining the efficiency of release bindings. A heel release check is being de-

TABLE IV. Age groups

Age (Years)	Number	Injury (Per Cent)	Number of Skiers (Per Cent)
0 to 6	17	2	1
7 to 12	199	24	8
13 to 17	236	29	16
18 to 21	172	21	11
22 to 30	117	14	35
31 to 40	55	7	22
Over 40	22	3	7
TOTAL	818		

114

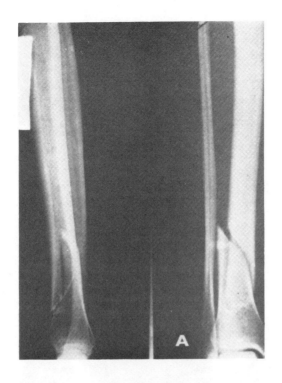

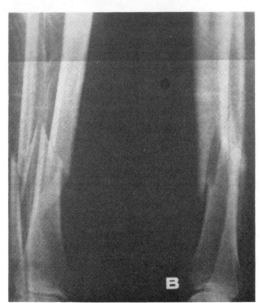

FIGURE 6. (A) Spiral fracture stable although oblique. (B) Unstable spiral fracture with fracture of fibula.

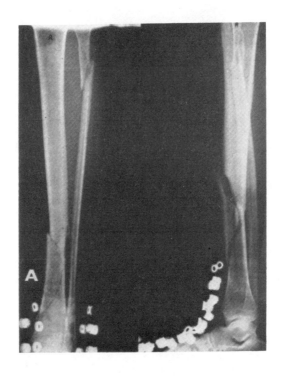

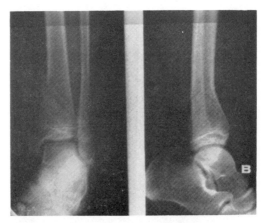

FIGURE 7. (A) Comminuted spiral fracture. (B) Boot-top fracture of tibia and fibula.

TABLE V. Experience

Times Skied	Number	Per Cent
First time	83	12
2 to 5 times	71	11
6 months to 1 year	143	21
1 to 2 years	152	23
2 to 3 years	84	12
3 to 5 years	88	13
Over 5 years	55	8
TOTAL	676	

veloped. An example of one prototype is shown in Figure 9B.

We checked the bindings with a small hand "release check" on a group of injured skiers who stated that their bindings did not release (Table VII). It is interesting that almost half of these were found to be adjusted improperly, particularly in the adult group. In three instances no release at all could be obtained because of faulty installation or faulty bindings. Eight cases were interesting in that the binding released easily and within the so-called normal limits to one side, but was definitely abnormal in its release to the other side. This happened to the woman, whose x-ray film of a comminuted spiral fracture was shown in Figure 7B. She had been skiing several times and had fallen to the right each time with the bindings releasing. Feeling that her bindings were well set, she was skiing harder and took a sudden turn to the left. As she twisted uphill, the edge caught and she felt her tibia snap as she fell to the ground. Checking her bindings showed that the release was set to the left 100 per cent heavier than compared to the right side which was properly set for her weight and skiing ability.

Some of the bindings for 120-pound people, who are just getting out of the beginner stages, were found to be set for releases equivalent to what would be

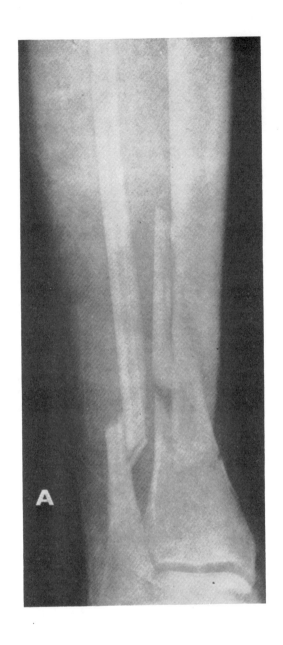

FIGURE 8. (A and B) Boot-top fractures of tibia and fibula.

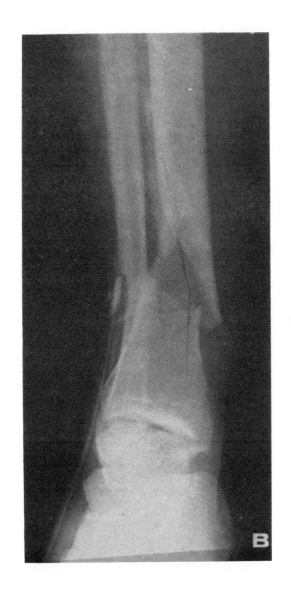

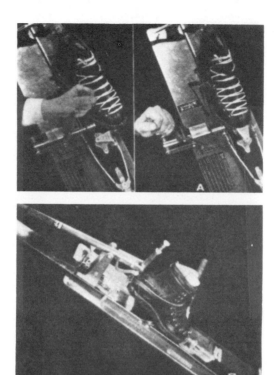

FIGURE 9. Testing mechanisms. (A) Pressure against side of boot building up tension until toe release effected. (B) Heel release check.

needed by an expert or racer weighing over 200 pounds.

This is not a critical adjustment in that Mr. Lipe believes that if the bindings are designed, manufactured, installed, and adjusted properly, there can be a margin of 20 per cent in the reading without the skier being inconvenienced by the bindings being too loose or too tight.

Conclusion

The subject of ski injuries has been discussed with the intention of making every one aware of the possibility of safety in skiing. Incidence, types of ski injuries, causes, and some modalities of prevention have been covered.

TABLE VI. Varying conditions of weight and skiing ability

Weight Without Ski Equipment (Pounds)	Beginner Novice	Advanced Novice	Inter-mediate	Advanced Inter-mediate	Expert	Racer
40 to 49	3	4	5	6	7	8
50 to 59	4	5	6	7	8	9
60 to 69	5	6	6	7	8	9
70 to 79	6	6	7	8	9	10
80 to 89	6	7	8	9	9	10
90 to 99	7	8	9	9	10	11
100 to 109	7	8	9	10	10	11
110 to 119	8	9	10	10	11	12
120 to 129	8	9	10	11	11	12
130 to 139	8	9	10	11	12	13
140 to 149	9	10	11	12	12	13
150 to 159	9	10	11	12	13	14
160 to 169	10	11	12	12	13	14
170 to 179	10	11	12	13	14	15
180 to 189	10	11	12	13	14	15
190 to 199	11	12	13	14	15	16
200 to 209	11	12	13	14	15	16
210 to 219	12	13	14	15	16	17
220 to 229	12	13	14	15	16	17
230 to 239	12	13	14	15	16	18

TABLE VII. Injured skiers whose bindings did not release at time of injury

Type of Injury	Under 16	Over 16 Male	Over 16 Female
Sprain of foot or ankle	8	3	2
Sprain of knee	2	8	5
Fracture of foot or ankle	1	2	2
Fracture of tibia or fibula	16	5	4
TOTALS	27	18	13

The skiing injury itself is considered only as a torsional type of injury to the lower extremities, which is, of course, peculiar to this sport.

Throughout New York State and in adjacent states, skiing is possible for approximately five months of the year. As orthopedists we will be confronted with both the local injuries and the aftercare and follow-up of more distant injuries to the musculoskeletal system. In addition, however, we are often asked for advice regarding equipment for many types of sports. With the increased popularity of skiing and other winter sports, we will have to be increasingly knowledgeable in this area.

References

1. Erskine, L. A.: The mechanisms involved in skiing injuries, Am. J. Surg. **97**: 667 (1959).
2. Ellison, A. E., Carroll, R. E., Haddon, W., Jr., and Wolf, M.: Skiing injuries. Clinical study, Pub. Health Rep. **77**: 985 (1962).
3. Leidholt, J. D.: Biomechanics of ankle injuries in skiing as related to release bindings, S. Clin. North America **43**: 363 (1963).
4. Dimond, J. H.: Isolated displaced fracture of posterior facet of talus, J. Bone & Joint Surg. **43-A**: 275 (1951).
5. Judd, W. R., and Hendryson, I. E.: Sitzmarks or Safety, Denver National Ski Patrol System, Inc., 1960.
6. Earle, A. S., Moritz, J. R., Saviers, G. B., and Ball, J. D.: Ski injuries, J.A.M.A. **180**: 285 (1962).
7. Wilson, C. L.: Fracture centers are urged for location in ski areas, Med. Tribune, December 23, 1964.
8. Lipe, G.: Personal communication.
9. Ellison, A.: Ski Magazine, February 1963.

Safety in a Release Binding

RICHARD TUCKER, M.D.

GORDON C. LIPE

Since the advent of modern skiing by Hannes Scheneider in the early part of this century, skiing has progressed to the sport we know today. At the present time, approximately two million individuals are exposed to the hazards of skiing. This does not include the occasional skier, but rather those who devote at least 15 days to this sport during the winter. During the past 20 years we have witnessed an exceedingly rapid growth of the skiing fraternity. This is due to the revolutionary new skiing techniques in addition to the marked improvement in equipment and increased leisure time.

Concomitant with the rise of skiing popularity is the parallel increase in awareness of skiing accidents.

The incidence of ski injuries is a real and provocative problem. The record needs facts. Part of the problem is that by nature of their location most ski resorts do not lend themselves to compiling adequate records.

The first leader in care and prevention of ski injuries was the National Ski Patrol System. This was started by Minot Dole in 1939 and has consisted of voluntary efforts by skiers themselves who freely give of their time to belong to this patrol.

During the past few years both Mt. Snow, Vermont, and Sun Valley, Idaho, by nature of their location and local medical facilities have found a ski injury incidence of 5.9 and 7.4 per 1,000 skiers, respectively. If we adjust these figures upward slightly to account for the injured skier who does not report his injury locally, we find that the actual incidence of ski injuries is in the neighborhood of about 8 per 1,000 skiers. This is not the 10% or (100/1,000 skiers) reported by the *Life* and *Time* articles of a few years back. It has been found that of the 8/1,000 ski injuries about 35% are fractures. Sprains account for about 45% with the remainder of the injuries consisting of wounds, freezing, snow blindness, and other minor injuries.

Cause of Injury

It is known that while only 25% of the skiers are between the ages of 13 and 21, they yield over 50% of the injuries. Females have a larger percentage of accidents than males and account for a much smaller proportion of the actual skiers. Over 64% of the injuries occur in skiers with less than two years of experience. The longer one skis and the more lessons he has had, the less accident prone he becomes.

To ski is to risk an element of injury. As in all problems of prevention, once an individual is aware that there is a problem, we have made a great step forward. In the final analysis it is the attitude of the skier that will determine the extent of decrease in the incidence of ski injuries.

Conditioning

Skiing safety depends upon *conditioning— 50%, control, judgment and courtesy—30%, and equipment—20%.* Skiing is a vigorous sport, often carried out in a difficult climate. It requires strength, coordination, sharp reflexes and endurance. Metabolic studies have shown that the average skier on a mountain expends the amount of energy used in running the mile. Obviously, sedentary and poorly coordinated individuals should

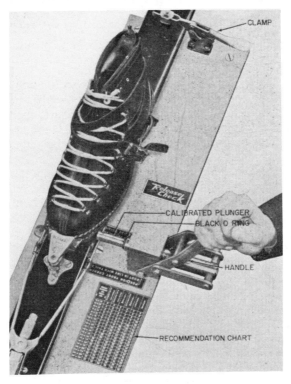

Figure 1

The entire Release Check Unit measures 3 ft. long by 9 in. wide. Plate is heavy duty aluminum complete with clamps to hold ski in place, spring loaded gauge with lever, recommendation chart and simple operating instructions. Unit is portable or may be mounted on a bench or on a wall if bench space is at a premium.

not attempt skiing. If one wishes to ski, one should continue some vigorous, year-around activity such as running, playing tennis and handball or similar activity. Golf is not a skiing conditioner.

Control

Control involves technical know-how as well as judgment. Skiing is a thrilling, yet risk-taking sport, thus one should prepare himself with as much technical know-how as possible. There is no substitute for lessons. Statistics bear this out.

The more lessons one has had, the less likely that injuries will occur. Courtesy involves *avoidable injuries*. Regard for your fellow skier is an extremely important factor, not only to him but to others. Practice the "golden rule" on the slopes as well as in daily life.

There is no question that the incidence of ski injuries could be remarkably reduced if the foregoing factors were kept in mind by all skiers. The incidence could be cut even further if one's equipment is the best available. All of us at one time or another ski near the limit of our ability in order to taste the exhilaration of skiing fast and this presents the possibility of injury.

Equipment

Last year a new device for checking release binding effectiveness was introduced. This unit was developed by a consulting engineer, who became concerned with the increase in incidence of ski injuries. During the past five years this intrepid young man has put a considerable amount of time and effort into investigating the causes of ski injuries and their prevention.

From his thorough investigations have come many new facts relative to how we ski and the cause of ski injuries. This study has resulted in the introduction of a "Release Check Unit." Actually there are two different units, one to check the toe release and the other to check the heel release. The devices are simple to use, and provide reliable results for setting both the toe and heel releases (Figure 1).

Complacency within the skiing industry, in the form of improper installation, added to the lack of knowledge and lack of understanding by the skier of his particular binding, have contributed immensely to the ineffectiveness of release bindings. The obvious result of this dilemma is an above normal rate of injury.

The release binding is ineffective, because we know by actual tests under controlled settings that very few bindings really qualify to do the job intended; even the best bindings must be properly installed and adjusted to be of any benefit.

126

Care of Bindings

Releasing the Freeze

One of the general beliefs pertaining to binding problems is icing up or freezing of the toe unit. Tests show that freezing will occur if a warm, wet ski is taken from the repair shop into cold air and used without breaking the unit loose and drying the parts.

Silicone Spray

The best preventive for any icing is silicone spray which is available in small cans, or a light coating of silicone grease. It is not messy, since it is transparent, and it also solves the problem of corrosion due to ·the salts used on highways which attack the dissimilar metals of a binding during transporting on the ski rack.

Aligning the Ski Boot

Notching the Boot

Notching of boots, where required, to engage the teeth of many of the toe units is extremely critical, and must be perfect to ensure the same release pressure left and right on the same ski. If one notch is deeper than the other, the binding will be out of balance and will cause inadvertent releases in one direction and a possible fracture in the other. Fifty per cent of bindings requiring a notch showed differences between left and right of 20% to 50%.

The Toe

The toe units must be mounted in line with the ski and boot centerline. If it is cocked, the forward pressure of the cable spring or heel closing spring unbalances the unit to one side, causing different pressures from left to right (Figure 2).

The Ball of the Foot

Friction between the ball of the foot and the ski provides poor binding performance. The toe hold-down adjustment in evidence on most toe units is a built-in clamp screw. Clearance between the hold-down and the boot sole is vital and should be maintained as more boot curl becomes evident. If a boot tree is used, the need for this is

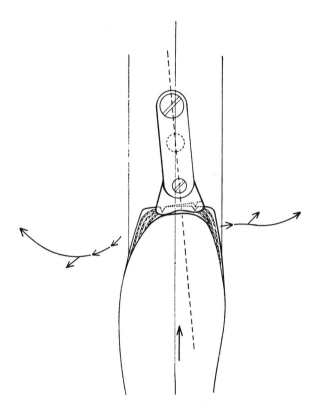

Figure 2

Toe units that require boot notching can function properly
only if the boots are notched properly. The boot is shown
on the ski and engaged with the toe piece. However, because the notches vary in depth, when the binding is
latched, the toe unit rotates slightly. The teeth have
"bottomed" in the notches and a partial release has taken
place. To release the boot to the left would require a
much higher force, since the boot has already gone over
center to the right.

minimized. Some will argue that edge control is
hampered if there is clearance here. Some bindings which provide for zero clearance by having
metal to metal contact between boot and ski, provide a more reliable release to be obtained through
lower coefficients of friction (Figure 3).

The Heel Release

The Rear Hook

If the low hitches or rear hooks through which
the cable passes are far enough back to pro-

128

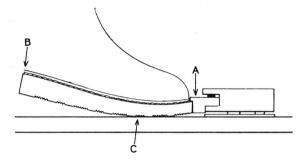

Figure 3

The toe hold down plate has been adjusted (Arrow A) so that the toe of the boot can be inserted easily, but when the skier stands on his skis and the heel is forced down (Arrow B), very high friction under the ball of the foot (Arrow C) may prevent a release. The height adjustment of the toe unit should be made with the heel down and loosened until there is no down pressure at the toe.

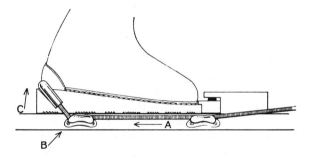

Figure 4a

Using this type of forward release mechanism, the cable must move to the rear (Arrow A) when the boot is lifted at the heel (Arrow C). High friction is evident at rear of low hitch (Arrow B) which in turn may prevent a release.

vide good heel hold-down and prevent side slip of the boot while edging, there is a good chance of negating the forward release due to the high friction of the cable passing through the hitches. Kinking of the cable because of these angles also results and causes release problems. If the low hitch is mounted one-half inch further forward than is usually recommended, this difficulty is obviated (Figures 4a and 4b).

129

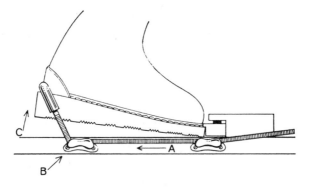

Figure 4b

In this view, the cable (Arrow A) has released and moved
back and trapped the skier in the binding, having achieved
only a 1½-inch movement (Arrow C) before being caught
by the cable. Moving the low hitches forward permits more
vertical movement and a better chance of a full release.
Note the severe cable angle at the rear of the side hitch
(Arrow B).

Dead Man Strap

Even if a release with a cable system is
achieved, there is no assurance that the cable will
come out of the boot groove. If you have not
fitted a "Dead Man Strap," which pulls the cable
off the boot, the resulting impact upon reaching
the end of the cable travel is sure to impart damaging inertia loads to, the achilles tendon. The
new Marker cable holder appears to be an effective device to free the cable in a fall, as well as the
usual Dead Man Strap.

Cable Tension

Cable tension causing forward pressure creates
tremendous friction at the pivot of the toe unit
which locks up the toe unit completely even if
the adjusting screw, spring, or ball are removed.
This will occur even if the unit previous to install-
ing the boot in the binding felt free to rotate in
both directions. These situations are common
and are difficult to solve if high cable tension or
spring tension is required for heel support.

130

The Toe Release

The ability of a toe unto to absorb shocks is a big asset. Many of these shock loads are high but intermittent and do not necessarily demand release. Nonflexible toe units require much higher settings to prevent inadvertent releases than the flexible units. Some impact type of nonflexible toe units require settings above the pressure which may be considered safe for slow twist release to hold the skier for normal skiing. Certain bindings are better for the beginner, while others should be used only by the expert. Special women's and children's bindings also are available.

Protruding Screws

Screws and nails protruding from boots and skis may cause some mysterious accidents, especially when the binding is in proper adjustment. The release may occur, but if the screws or nails hamper the full release, they can cause the injury that is otherwise unexplainable.

Negative Camber

Although not too common, our records indicate injuries have been received as a result of bindings increasing in tension at the toe due to negative camber (that is the up-bowing of the ski at the tip and tail), causing the boot to become "squeezed" into place. These do not use front cable bindings needing strong tension.

Which Safety Strap?

Common sense dictates the use of some method which can prevent injuries to others from a runaway ski. A single strap is better than nothing, but the resulting "windmill" of the ski after a release can inflict some serious lacerations.

The Arlberg Strap

The "Arlberg" strap or double strap which reduces "windmilling" is better than the single strap. A warning is in order, however, to those whose Arlberg straps are attached directly to the skis under the boot. MAKE SURE THEY DO NOT INTERFERE WITH THE BOOT. Do not tighten the strap as a long-thong, because you may negate both releases. Be certain the Arlberg

131

strap is attached just ahead of the rear cable holder.

The Ski Halter

The ski halter or ski stop lever, which forces the ski to stop when the binding releases, is the best solution to the problem. The ski does not continue down the hill but remains nearby. At the same time, it is not beating and cutting the skier.

Mixing the Bindings

Mixing the toe and heel brands is not good practice, as a general rule. In some instances, however, it does work. The Nevada toe used with Look cables, the Grand Prix Heel or the Look Turnable work fine. You may not get a release of a Nevada toe if you use the Geze Turnable, because the travel of the Geze Turnable is restricted and may not swing far enough for a complete release.

The Release Check Instrument

The release check and the heel check devices simulate the action required of a boot in a release, and measure the load required to perform the release. Static rather than dynamic loading is used, because it is the slow twist or low inertia condition which puts the greatest demand on the binding during the release period. The chart which recommends the various settings for various individuals represents the maximum allowable settings for safety in slow pressure build-up before the release occurs. By using this method of testing we can see the problems occur exactly, or as nearly so as possible, as they would occur in actual skiing. Numbers below maximum are the rule rather than the exception with the better bindings, since greater safety is obtained with an even greater margin of retention than with the poorer bindings at higher settings.

Comments

Accidents will happen even if all the mechanical problems are corrected. They cannot all be prevented. Fractures occur when the release of the binding is not even a factor. Physical conditioning for the sport, coupled with common sense

132

judgment of the skier's ability to handle conditions and careful inspection of equipment, are still the best deterrent to injury. Some loads which occur to the leg, which we term "combined loads," cannot be adjusted for and no binding on the market can prevent injury in these cases. We do not have all the answers, but we certainly know much more about the problems which cause bindings to become inoperable than ever before. We know what has to be done to eliminate most of them, and despite the fact that there are only a few really good binding designs, we have been able, under our IBM control, to reduce the accident rate within the control by 50%.

As better binding designs become available, as the shops become more aware of their responsibility in mounting the bindings, and as the skiing public becomes better educated about binding operation, we hope the accident rate will be reduced even further.

Conclusions

1. Stay in top physical condition. Continue with some vigorous year-round conditioning program.

2. Use judgment—do not overestimate your ability.

3. Be courteous.

4. Beginners should go to ski school and stay there until well past the snowplow stage. They should avoid "free" lessons from well meaning but otherwise unqualified persons.

5. Be alert at all times, particularly on lower slopes where traffic is heavy and collision danger is high.

6. Use release bindings. Know your release binding adjustment and check your release binding daily.

7. Be sure release bindings are mounted properly.

8. Avoid use of straps which allow ski to snap back or too much play so that they may whirl around. Both of these types are a major cause of lacerations.

9. Once bindings are adjusted, do not switch skis. Skis should be marked right and left, so that the same boot goes on the same ski each time.

Needs for Diving Accident Information

H. William Gillen, MD

Both PROFESSIONAL and amateur diving with compressed gas sources cause a number of medical hazards and accidents. Whenever a person uses a gas mixture under pressure as a breathing gas source he is vulnerable to indirect toxicologic effects of some of the gases themselves (oxygen toxicity, inert-gas narcosis, and carbon-dioxide poisoning) as well as to the toxic effects of contaminants of the gas supply such as carbon monoxide; he is exposed to the hazards of decompression sickness, air embolism, explosive decompression (blow-up) and drowning.

The divers, their employers, physicians, and insurance carriers are all concerned with the existence of these accidents and hazards, their frequency, treatment, and prevention. Appropriate treatment of each problem often requires both specialized training and experience, and specialized facilities such as medically supervised recompression chambers. Planning the prevention or treatment of any of these accidents or hazards requires valid information about their incidence and relative frequency. This information is almost completely lacking outside of the military and then only if military diving *per se* is under consideration. The need for data on diving accidents, underwater hazards, and underwater accidents associated with the act of diving from non-military sources is tremendous. There can be no planning by employers without it; community planning by public health authorities cannot be started on a reasonable basis; no regulations controlling or qualifying the act of diving by amateurs or the profession of diving by commercial divers can be contemplated intelligently without the information that can only be obtained from conscientious, continuous, and correlated reporting of these accidents.

Several attempts have been made to overcome this important deficiency in data. Unfortunately, very little assistance has been obtained from possible sources of the needed information. Concerted effort and informed action by the divers, their employers, local health authorities, workmen's compensation boards, and insurance carriers could result in data accumulation that would be of benefit to all concerned, particularly to the divers, themselves. Commercial diving costs could be reduced if accidents could be prevented or if, when they occur unavoidably, proper treatment were available. Many persons could be alive today if this were so, just as many who have been irrevocably crippled as a result of diving accidents and hazards could be leading normal, healthy, productive lives if both prevention and proper treatment were available.

(The Committee on Man's Underwater Activities of the Marine Technology Society has initiated a study of the reporting of diving and underwater accidents and would appreciate comments from all interested persons, agencies or companies.)

The Need for Practical Methods of Presymptomatic Bubble Detection

JON LINDBERGH

In a display at this Symposium there is the figure of a diver with bubbles coursing through his veins. If you step on the lever, you can hear the sound of those bubbles as they pass through a Doppler flowmeter. This is not just an abstract demonstration. What you hear is actually the taped sound of bubbles as they were going through the veins of an experimental animal. We can be pretty sure those same bubbles and those same sounds would be in the veins of a man in similar circumstances, when he was being decompressed too rapidly.

This research was developed at the Virginia Mason Research Center, Seattle Washington, in an attempt to find a means to identify bubbles in the system before they develop the symptoms of decompression sickness or "the bends." Have we merely a curiosity, something which a scientist looks at and is excited about because it is new? Or will it mean something practical to us as we try to work deeper in the ocean and do more? To find the answer we must begin by looking back into history. The earliest divers held their breath, grabbed a rock and headed for the bottom of the sea. They harvested sponges, pearls, and other marine life from depths to 100 feet. There is a limit to how long a man can hold his breath and that limit is far less than it takes for significant nitrogen to be absorbed into the system and give trouble with bends.

In the Eighteenth century, an Englishman by the name of Augustus Siebe developed a metal helmet with a window in the front and a canvas suit bolted on underneath. He attached a hose and had a couple of men on deck to pump down air. With the Siebe helmet, underwater man was no longer limited to the time he could hold his breath. He could stay as long as the deck hands were willing to crank the pump. He was able to see and move about as he wished. For the first time he could really accomplish useful work. Inevitably he began to probe deeper and stay longer. Problems developed. A diver would ascend from a long deep dive and complain of violent pain. Sometimes he fell to the deck contorted in agony. The dread "bends" had been discovered.

Another Englishman, J. B. S. Haldane, found that the nitrogen in air is forced into the bloodstream and body tissues by increased pressure under water. If one returns to normal pressure too quickly, the nitrogen does not dissolve back out, but forms bubbles, much as in a champagne bottle when the cork is popped. Haldane established a procedure whereby divers can come up in a series of slow calculated stages, rather than one quick jump. The nitrogen, thus, has time to exit peacefully.

Since the time of Haldane, more sophisticated tables have been worked out. The U.S. Navy, over a period of some years, has developed a set of tables which are doctrine for air diving in this country and many other areas. The Navy tables are good, but by no means 100% effective. Tables are designed around time and depth; the development of bends varies with many other factors. First, perhaps, is the individual himself. Different people are susceptible in different degrees. Some violate the tables to a certain extent without appearing to have trouble. Others need to be more conservative. I am reminded of the chief diver on a sewer outfall job in San Diego. He would always make the first dive in the morning. Then he would go in the decompression chamber, stay all day long, and come out with the last diver at night. By so doing, he was able to get through the day without symptoms.

The physical and perhaps mental condition of an individual affects susceptibility. Some days you get bent — other days you do not — doing the same thing at the same depth. I have never, personally, been able to pick out the more susceptible days. I have been bothered by mild bends after plenty of sleep, yet 24 hours later, exhausted, had no trouble at all. Your degree of physical work has an effect, as well as the water temperature. Previous cases of severe bends appear to be significant, perhaps also shocks such as might be induced by an underwater explosion in the general area. Or simply the chance formation of a bubble.

Sometimes "the bends" is merely painful, but often it can be serious. On the same job where the chief diver was spending all day in the tank, there was also a fairly young diver. Eighteen successive dives were made on a structure in 210 feet of water. On the nineteenth dive, the young man spent 27 minutes on the bottom. At 60 feet, on his ascent, he complained that he "didn't feel right." At 30 feet, he was dizzy, and approaching unconsciousness. He was immediately surfaced and recompressed on "Table IV." A day later he died, in spite of the best efforts of the top submarine medical officers in San Diego. In the critique of the accident afterward, nobody could give any clear-cut reasons why this man was hit fatally after the previous 18 uneventful dives.

With increasing depth, air has become impractical and divers use helium-oxygen breathing mixtures. Helium-oxygen has different decompression characteristics from air, and new tables were needed. At first this meant the Navy's helium partial pressure tables. Adapting Navy helium tables to commercial operations was a matter of trial and error during the first years. We picked a table according to the rules, and if somebody ached on the way up, we simply went to a more conservative table next time. On my own first helium dive, to about 250 feet, I came up by the book. At the 50 foot stop there was slight pain in my elbows. At 40 feet, it was a little worse. I still was not quite sure whether this meant trouble or just a normal ache. On deck, there was no question — trouble!

We also felt that the use of pure oxygen during the latter stages of water decompression, as per Navy doctrine, was not particularly safe with our equipment. We had had one accident from an apparent oxygen convulsion at 40 foot depth. This may have been unusual, but we worried about it and decided to substitute air for oxygen. After a 380 foot helium dive using air instead of oxygen for decompression, my elbows again objected strenuously. The next man said that when he reached the deck, he saw three doors on the decompression tank. He felt he had better get in fast before the number increased and his chances of hitting the right one went down.

We were not too pleased with this state of affairs, so we went to people like Capt. Behnke and Dr. Schreiner for their advice on how to improve the situation. These men took all the data they could find and worked it into formulas. They programmed the formulas into computers, which produced tables calculated to avoid the bends. But, the only way to really check a table out is to make a dive on it, first in a chamber and then in the water. Those check dives were a time of frustration. Someone would be hit by the bends. The affected man was treated and the new data went back into the computer. On the next dive it would be the same story. Sometimes the hits occurred on parts of the decompression profile which had proven safe on a dozen previous ascents, including some by the man hit. This continued for months! The problem was not so simple as we had anticipated.

We now have tables which are fairly effective, but to avoid all accidents, it would be necessary to take an excessive amount of ascent time. Dr. Schreiner has said that to be entirely safe for a one hour dive at 300 feet, we should take perhaps 70 hours of decompression. If we are willing to accept more risk, we can come up in ten hours. In practice that is what we do. Industry cannot afford those additional 60 hours.

Let us digress a moment and examine the problem of safety. It is sometimes stated that safety is paramount — that there is no justification for coming up in ten hours if a risk is involved. But that is not the approach we take in most phases of our lives. Look at the automobile. If we were willing to drive at ten miles an hour on a highway, there would not be very many fatal accidents. However, we drive 70 miles an hour and lose 50,000 people a year on the highways. We must think it worth the risk — that it simply is not acceptable in this civilization to travel at ten miles per hour. In the diving industry, the same thing applies. We cannot afford to take 70 hours to come up from each dive. With our present knowledge, it is necessary to take certain chances.

However, if there were some means to detect incipient cases of bends in a diver prior to symptoms, we could monitor the actual state of decompression much more accurately. We can do this, to a certain extent, with pain. When a man hurts, you slow down. This would be all right if all that was involved was a little pain, but pain is not all that is involved. Sometimes the bubble causing the difficulty is in the brain or the central nervous system. More than pain can result, even permanent damage. You will recall the aseptic bone necrosis described by Capt. Behnke.

If the bubbles could be detected *before* they cause pain, *before* they threaten bone necrosis or central nervous system difficulties, then the man could be brought up according to the development of pre-symptomatic bubbles. We are looking at a situation where the ten hour decompression can always be used without the present risk. If on a certain day or under certain conditions a man cannot come up in ten hours but needs 15, then we can react before dangerous symptoms occur.

How are we going to spot the bubbles early enough? Perhaps with a transcutaneous Doppler flowmeter, one which you put over your veins, or perhaps a sonic detector will prove best. The use of such instruments may be difficult for surface based helmet divers decompressing in the water, but for very deep diving, surface based divers are no longer used. Modern deep diving systems allow a man to decompress inside a submersible decompression chamber or mating deck decompression chamber where it is dry. Conditions are easily adaptable to simple instrumentation.

With submersible decompression chambers we can go much deeper than with the old equipment. It may. turn out that a number of other gas mixtures beside helium-oxygen are advantageous. We have even looked at pharmaceuticals and other novel means of improving decompression. What this means is that there will be multiplicity of decompression profiles — of tables — that must be investigated. Presymptomatic bubble detection will vastly simplify and speed up the development of these tables, it will also enable us to use them with confidence in the field.

The Role of the Team Physician and Trainer

THE TEAM PHYSICIAN
AND THE LAW

A. A. SAVASTANO, M.D.

In this lawsuit conscious age suits claiming negligence against school officials, coaches, trainers, and physicians have become a reality and are on the increase. Those who are serving as team physicians will do well to take every precaution to avoid becoming directly involved as defendants in tort liability cases. The concepts expressed in the succeeding pages should be thoroughly understood by physicians who become responsible for the medical supervision and treatment of athletes.

A careful pre-season medical evaluation has become an integral part of an athlete's preparation for participation in sports. The principal object of the evaluation is to furnish each athlete with the medical guidance best suited to his special desires and capabilities. Health guidance does not cease with the pre-season medical evaluation. The athlete whenever possible should receive health guidance throughout the season. Assurance of medical services for all athletic contests where injuries may be anticipated should be an important provision in a school's or college's athletic program. Other provisions should include the privilege for physicians to handle on-site injuries under desirable conditions, pre-arranging emergency medical care at practice sessions when a physician is not in attendance, and the establishment of procedures and policies that provide the best medical protection for the athlete. Colleges and universities in most cases have no problem maintaining adequate medical supervision by drawing from the student health services or from consultants. On the other hand high schools as a rule do not enjoy the medical luxury that colleges and universities enjoy; consequently, arrangements have to be made with private physicians. The secondary schools in most cases get medical coverage by seeking the help of local medical societies.

WHAT IS A TEAM PHYSICIAN?

The Committee on the Medical Aspects of Sports of the American Medical Association states that "the title *Team Physician* denotes a physician who is vested by the school with authority to make medical judgments relating to the participation and supervision of students in school sports. Without such a categorical designation of responsibility, there cannot exist the continuing medical assistance the athlete deserves."

The Committee further states "Having accepted the responsibility of acting in behalf of the school, the team physician faces a dual responsibility of ensuring: (1) That the athlete is not deprived unnecessarily of the opportunity to participate if an injury or other clinical condition is not potentially serious and does not interfere with the player's performance; and conversely (2) That the student's future in athletics and in life is not jeopardized by unwarranted eligibility for a particular sport or by premature return to competition in any sport after injury or illness."

The team physician must have the full and complete final say in decisions pertaining to medical eligibility of athletic participation. He must have authority to obtain consultations if such are needed.

145

WHY IS PRE-PARTICIPATION MEDICAL EVALUATION NECESSARY?

There are many reasons why this is of utmost importance. Chief among which are the following: (1) To determine the health status of prospective athletes prior to their being exposed to participation in competition; (2) To promote optimum health and fitness; (3) To recommend or arrange for further evaluation and treatment of remediable problems; (4) To advise atypical candidates as to sports which for them would provide suitable activity; and (5) To restrict from participation those whose physical limitations present undue risk.

Health examinations of prospective athletes may be accomplished in several ways. The prospective athlete may be examined by the family physician on an individual basis or he can be examined by the school or team physician if one is available. If the above are not available, then arrangements can be made with local medical societies. In order to allow for consultations and treatment if abnormalities are found, the medical evaluation should not be for a specific sport, but for all sports available in that community or school. It is to be remembered that not all sports are contact sports. It may be proper for an athlete to engage in one sport, but not in another.

There has been much comment regarding the team physician and possible or probable legal implications in his work. Physicians should be cautioned to avoid giving any guarantee that it would be safe for a candidate to participate in a given sport. In addition the physician should not undertake medical treatment without the parents prior consent, express or implied, except for first aid or emergency care which is reasonably necessary to save life or limb. Beyond these considerations, if the physician conforms to the standards of good medical practice in his community there is no reason why medical supervision of any athletic team entails risks of legal liability any greater than in any other area of medical practice.

A joint statement on the legal liability of team physicians in January, 1966 by the Law Department and the Committee on the Medical Aspects of Sports of the American Medical Association reads as follows: "There appears to be no reason why the risks of legal liability for a physician who

146

undertakes the medical supervision and care of members of a school athletic team should be any different from that of a physician in any other branch of practice. In fact, careful examination of reported court decisions and a survey of attorneys for the state medical societies has disclosed very few suits arising out of the medical supervision of school athletic teams or the treatment of injured student athletes at the scene of the injury. Likewise, no record has been found of other cases in which a physician has been sued because of emergency medical care given at the scene of any accident.

"A team physician should conform to the standards of good medical practice in his community. If he undertakes to determine the fitness of a team member to participate in athletic activities, he should be careful not to give any guarantee or assurances that it will be safe for the team member to so participate. It is better for him to state that there appears to be no medical reason why this boy should not participate. Institutions sponsoring athletic teams are urged to require prior written approval from parents of a minor, or the player himself if he has obtained his majority for necessary emergency treatment by the team physician as need may arise. Such a practice, it is felt, would make it clear that the team physician was carrying out an appropriate function in providing emergency treatment on the field or in the training room."

RELEASES AND WAIVERS

Some college team physicians in their pre-season medical examinations occasionally find certain physical defects which normally should be disqualifying. However, in these situations the college team physician is told that the athlete has been participating in practically all sports since grade school. In these situations the coach, the athlete, or even the parents may not be able to understand why the physician considers such defects disqualifying, the parents, therefore, offer to sign a release. The defects most commonly found include loss of a paired organ, history of convulsive disorders, repeated episodes of concussion of the brain, and certain joint or musculo-skeletal problems. Since most athletes are minors, the physician may ask:

1) Is a statement signed by the parents to re-

linquish any future claims against the individual coach, trainer, or physician of any value?

2) What is the liability of the physician if he does not qualify the athlete to participate, but does nothing to prevent the school department from allowing the athlete to compete?

Generally speaking the parent has no authority to release future claims on behalf of the child. It is to be remembered that the statute of limitations does not begin until the child has become of age. The same thing may be said regarding a release by the minor himself. It is recommended that, when the team physician deems an individual unfit to participate in any given sport or sports, he should in writing inform the parents, the athlete, and the school or college as to his findings. If the physician finds that contrary to his recommendations the boy is participating in sports, he will do well to write again stating his objections to continued participation.

The National Safety Council reports that 67 per cent of all school jurisdiction accidents involving boys, and 59 per cent involving girls occur in physical education and recreation.

WHAT IS NEGLIGENCE?

Negligence is failure to act as a prudent physician would under the same circumstances. Negligence can consist of inaction as well as of action. If one fails to do something expected of him by the law, he can be deemed negligent. Likewise, doing something contrary to what the law expects can also be considered negligence. The mere fact of an accident does not imply that the physician is liable, no matter how serious the injury is. If there is no negligence, there is no liability. However, if an injury is sustained by an athlete because of the physician's negligence, the physician may be liable for it.

CASE EXAMPLE

Welch v. Dunsmuir Joint Union High School District, 326, *P. 2d* 633 (*Calif.* 1958)

During a pre-season high school football scrimmage, the plaintiff — the quarterback on one of the teams — attempted a "quarterback sneak."

After being tackled, the plaintiff continued to lie

on his back. The coach of the high school, suspecting that the plaintiff might have suffered an injury to the neck, had him take hold of his hands to determine if he were able to grip, which he was able to do at that time.

The player was now carried off the field by eight other players, allegedly without anyone ordering the moving. There was conflicting testimony as to whether or not a doctor, who was admittedly present, examined the plaintiff before he was moved to the sidelines. The only undisputed medical testimony was that the plaintiff is a permanent quadriplegic — caused by damage to the spinal cord in his neck. It was the medical witness's opinion that the injury to the spinal cord took place during the removal of the player from the field without the use of a stretcher. Medical testimony brought out that the failure to use a stretcher was improper medical practice. It was also brought out by the medical witness that the player's ability to grip things with his hand while on the field was proof that the damage had not been done by the tackle, but had occurred afterwards.

The court felt that the evidence indicated that both the doctor and the coach were negligent in the removal of the plaintiff from the field to the sidelines — the coach for failing to wait for the doctor and allowing the plaintiff to be moved, and the doctor for failing to act promptly after the plaintiff's injury.

Judgment — $206,804.00 plus interest and *costs*.

MISMATCHING OF CONTESTANTS

It has been reported that in Oregon in 1961 an inexperienced uncoordinated 15 year old 140 pound high school male freshman was allowed to engage in an interschool football game against a superior team of large experienced boys. This boy allegedly had not received proper instruction and broke his neck. The court ruled that a coach is negligent and fails to take reasonable care of his players when he permits such students to play without proper or adequate instruction.

This case raises several interesting points. The problem of mismatching contestants can become a serious one. In New York a court found negligence because of mismatching of heights and weights in a supervised soccer game. One student was kicked in the head, and another suffered a serious injury.

On the other hand there was no negligence in another New York case where a student was injured in wrestling, which was part of the Physical Education Course. Here the activity was under the supervision of a competent person who had approved the voluntary matching of two boys, after comparison of weights and after watching them wrestle together. A California court saw no negligence where seventh and eighth grade teams played touch football and participants had been selected according to skill, and had been properly instructed, and were experienced.

It must be remembered that educational institutions and persons connected with school sports programs become subject to legal liabilities under certain circumstances for injuries occuring during sports participation. This liability in general is established through what in legal language is termed "tort liability." This is the type of liability for personal injuries allegedly caused through a defendant's negligence. According to James S. Fewrig, M.D.: "In order to succeed any such action in tort involves the proof of four essential elements, namely,

1) That the defendant owes a duty to avoid unreasonable risks to others.
2) That the defendant fails to observe that duty.
3) That the failure to observe the duty causes the damage which occurred.
4) That damage did in fact occur to the plaintiff and that the nature and probable extent of the damage are established proofs."

It has become the trend of the times to expand the areas in which tort liability is applied and also to increase the size of tort awards. It is also obvious that the tort case has become a reality in the realm of sports and that these cases are increasing in frequency.

Suits claiming negligence against team physicians, coaches, trainers, and school officials have increased to a marked degree. Doctors serving as team physicians may find themselves involved in legal action in one of two ways, either through tort liability or through direct malpractice suits. Tort cases may involve specifically educational institutions or include a number of defendants.

The team physician is usually involved either as a co-defendant or in a direct malpractice action.

In nearly all cases the plaintiff will argue that responsibility for the diagnosis and the treatment of sports injuries should not be the responsibility of coaches and trainers, but should be that of a physician. It is because of this premise that the team physician usually is the major defendant in practically all litigation cases. Regardless of the type of legal action instituted, either tort liability or malpractice, the principal charge which the team physician will have to defend is that of negligence on his part. The juries in these cases usually maintain that a patient-doctor relationship exists between the team physician and the members of the teams under his care. Many physicians serve gratis as "team doctors;" however, it becomes immaterial whether diagnosis or therapy are performed for a fee or gratis. Courts do not differentiate between charity and fee cases. There is an erroneous concept that team physicians who are employed by a state-owned education institution are immune to suit. It is also generally thought that one cannot sue the state unless the state accepts the suit. Regardless of the position of the state in such matters, the physician enjoys absolutely no immunity from lawsuit even when in the employ of the state.

It is also interesting that the statute of limitations, which varies in the several states, is no safeguard against action by a minor, as he can withhold a suit for negligence until he reaches maturity, this in spite of the fact that in ordinary cases the statute of limitations extends to two years from the date of the discovery of the alleged wrong act. Although a trainer may have been probably responsible for the negligence, juries generally regard trainers as agents of the team physician, and negligence on their part is very often imputed to the physician.

Feuring states that liability problems arising from injuries sustained in sports are contingent upon factors which are encountered in private practice. They are based on the premise that there has been a failure to follow the standard procedures and the established methods for the treatment of an injury. The team physician should always conduct himself professionally just as if he were engaged in private practice. Liability suits can arise from many and varied types of negligence charges. Some of these accusations seem almost

151

petty; but, nevertheless, they can be the basis for an award.

Among situations which can be causes of action are the following: 1) Failure to recognize an injury; 2) Certification of a participant with known limitations for a sport; 3) Premature termination of treatment; 4) Failure to follow-up a case which is under treatment, as this may be construed as abandonment of treatment. When athletes terminate treatment before they are medically discharged, it would be wise for the physician to make a serious attempt to get these men to resume treatment; and 5) Failure to refer for consultation to qualified specialists; 6) Failure to explain preoperatively to both the parents and the injured any surgical procedures anticipated and the possible results of this surgery; 7) Promises or guarantees of full, excellent, or good recovery for any specific case; 8) Inadequate recovery in a case in which a new treatment has been tried without explaining same to patients or parents; 9) Failure to obtain x-ray studies of an area of trauma; 10) Failure to check a cast after its application for abnormal constriction or compression; 11) Failure to administer anti-tetanus drugs when indicated; 12) Failure to administer antibiotics when indicated; and 13) Failure to elicit allergic history before prescribing medication.

CONCLUSIONS

In order to reduce the incidence of tort-malpractice claims, it is well for a team physician to use good medical judgment, follow and control all sports injury cases, keep good medical records, be in complete control over injury cases, have good working relationships with trainers, keep parents of an injured athlete well informed, never promise complete cures, and not permit anybody to pressure him to allow a boy to play if the boy has not fully recovered from an injury. Finally, a team physician should always be covered by adequate malpractice insurance, either institutional or individual, or both.

REFERENCES

[1]Feurig J. S.: Legal Liabilities of Team Physicians. Student Med. 10:479, 1962

[2]Rosenfield, H. N.: Legal Liability for School Accidents. Remarks Made at the National Conference

on Accident Prevention in Physical Education, Athletics and Recreation, Washington, D.C., December 7, 1963

[3]Leibee, H. C.: Tort Liability for Injuries to Pupils. Campus Publishers, Ann Arbor, Michigan, 1965

[4]AMA Committee on the Medical Aspects of Sports: The Team Physician. Statement Issued September 1967

[5]AMA Law Department and Committee on the Medical Aspects of Sports: Joint Statement on the Legal Liability of Team Physicians, January 1966

The Physician in the Training Room

Allan J. Ryan, M.D.

● Success in rehabilitation of an athlete following an injury is related directly to the time interval which elapses before the beginning of treatment. Recent studies have clarified mechanisms of injury and pathology of lesions, enabling the sports physician to make more exact diagnoses and to orient therapy toward more specific goals. The selection of appropriate treatment is a medical responsibility, though the decision may be influenced by the trainer. Drug therapy and surgical treatment is utilized more frequently today than in the past for the severely injured joint. With the development of sports medicine as a medical specialty, some physicians are devoting full time to medical supervision and care of athletes. Close cooperation is essential between the trainer and the physician, which requires that the physician visit the training room on frequent occasions, not just at the time an athlete is injured.

Not too many years ago, the appearance of a physician in a training room for sports, except in the event of an injury to an athlete, was an unusual occurrence. Today, with the development of sports medicine as a medical specialty, many physicians are devoting full time to medical supervision and care of athletes. They work closely with athletic trainers in prevention and treatment of injuries, which requires their presence in quarters previously considered the sole domain of the trainer.

I shall confine my discussion of sports physicians' responsibilities to those which involve treatment of acute and chronic athletic injuries. It should be understood that the trainer has always worked under standing or specific orders from a physician. The big difference today is that the broad standing orders formerly given the trainer allowed him a great deal of latitude as to selection of treatment and its extent and duration; present developments in knowledge of new techniques in management of sports injuries have greatly limited the area covered by standing orders, necessitating closer cooperation between the trainer and physician.

Studies and repeated close observations by sports physicians have clarified mechanisms and pathology of lesions due to sports injuries, enabling more exact diagnosis and orientation of treatment towards more specific goals. A good example lies in the differentiation of many conditions formerly grouped under the term "shin splints." Previous failure to distinguish between these causes was undoubtedly responsible for many failures in treatment. Making a specific diagnosis in these cases in order to introduce rational treatment necessarily involves the physician since it is properly not the trainer's responsibility and not within his area of competence. The selection of appropriate treatment is also a medical responsibility, even though the decision may be shared with the trainer.

Drug therapy, formerly rarely necessary in the treatment of sports injuries except for application of linaments, is now frequently—some might say too frequently — employed. Whether or not the drug is given by mouth, it must be prescribed by the physician, and if by needle, it must be injected by the physician, since nurses are seldom found in training rooms except at the Olympic Games.

Surgical treatment is utilized more frequently today than in the past for the severely injured joint. Although during the past 15 years indications for urgent surgical treatment of acute joint injuries in athletes have become well recognized by orthopedic surgeons, following the lead of the great pioneer, Dr. Don O'Donoghue, diagnosis still presents a difficult problem. Immediate or early examination of the injury, followed by repeated observations in the first 24 to 48 hours, may be required. This means

Presented at the Twenty-Ninth Annual Assembly of the American Academy of Physical Medicine and Rehabilitation, Miami Beach, Florida, August 29, 1967.

that the physician must frequently visit the training room as well as the hospital.

The success of a program of rehabilitation following a sports injury is often related directly to the interval of time which elapses between the injury and the beginning of treatment. It depends also in great measure on the individualization of treatment, which involves cooperation between the trainer and the physician.

Assuming the presence of the usual facilities of a training room in a university or a professional sports arena, the physician and the trainer are faced with a number of possibilities for specific treatment of an acute or a chronic athletic injury. Some training rooms seem to rely on the theory that there is greater safety with much equipment and literally bristle with expensive apparatus. Other training rooms have a Spartan simplicity, apparently making hands do more than machines. I have not yet been able to establish any correlation between abundance or paucity of mechanical and electric equipment and the success of a rehabilitation program. The chief advantage which might be cited in favor of less equipment is that there are fewer opportunities offered for errors.

In the average high school, training rooms as described do not exist. The coach is also the trainer and the physician seldom appears except before and after games. Occasionally, in such settings one may find whirlpool baths, diathermy, and even ultrasonic apparatus. The qualifications of the coach to use this equipment, even under the supervision of the physician, who may know no more about its use than the coach, are open to question. It is not realistic to expect that many of our high schools in the near future will be able to employ a qualified trainer since few are available and the shortage has priced them out of the high school market.

In the well-equipped training room today one may expect to find machines which supply hot and cold packs, heat lamps, ultraviolet lamps, diathermy equipment of various kinds, ultrasonic apparatus, and various types of electrical stimulators. If there is not a separate room for exercise therapy, the training room will also have tables for resistive exercises, pulleys with weights, barbells, and other types of weight apparatus.

The increase in the use of ultrasonic therapy for soft-tissue lesions in athletes has been phenomenal since its introduction about twenty years ago. This growth has been brought about largely by the enthusiastic salesmanship of the companies manufacturing the equipment rather than because of the accumulation of therapeutic experience carefully documented and reported as to its beneficial effects.

At the present time therapeutic ultrasonic equipment is present in nearly every department of physical therapy, whether in clinic or hospital, in physicians' offices, and in athletic training rooms. Physical therapists, physicians and athletic trainers are using it, chiefly according to the instructions of the manufacturer, seldom as the only treatment but often in conjunction with diathermy, other heat applications, massage and exercise. Treatments for the most part are administered by technicians with only very general instructions from physicians as to the exact number and duration of treatments and type of therapy applied.

When trainers are questioned about their clinical use and observed results of ultrasound, their comments vary from the extreme enthusiasm of those who have found a wide range of usefulness in treatment of soft-tissue injuries with exceptionally good results to the indifference of others who reply that they use it because they think it is the thing to do but are not really convinced of its advantages and to the disillusionment of those who have abandoned its use but still have the machine.

At the University of Wisconsin the core of rehabilitation of the athlete is believed to lie in the maintenance of optimal muscle strength and endurance and of maximal flexibility and muscular coordination in the whole body. Efforts are directed toward these objectives as strength and mobilty are restored to an injured part as rapidly as possible. Conventional exercise therapy is employed to accomplish these aims with isometric, isotonic exercises and progressive resistance exercises. In conjunction with exercises, physical applications of cold, heat and electricity are utilized, though very selectively with a great deal of respect for what is not known about their effects.

I feel that the physicians and trainers who are working daily with athletes, who do not have the time, background, financial support or facilities to conduct basic research into the effects of physical means of treatment on acute, subacute and chronic soft-tissue lesions, are entitled to more information than they now have regarding what can be expected from such use and how such therapy should be used. I believe that the responsibility for providing this information rests upon the members of this organization either individually or collectively. When such information is available, we may still not do a great deal better than we are doing now as far as treatment of sports injuries is concerned, but we may avoid making some errors and wasting time, manpower and money in a shotgun approach which is predicated on the basis of our presently inadequate knowledge.

The Medical Aspects of

Professional Baseball

Jacob R. Suker, M.D.

The team physician for a professional baseball team is faced with a variety of medical problems on a daily basis. It is a unique and often times an exciting experience. On any given day he may be required to treat a sore throat, listen to the latest physiologic explanation for a batting slump, comment on the medical report of a player to be obtained in a trade or learn that his team has just concluded a series in a city that has an epidemic of encephalitis. During the season his potential patient pool consists of 25 players, 4 coaches and a manager from his own team and a like number from the visiting team. In addition to the major league teams, he is responsible for the medical care of four umpires and the administrative staff of the organization. He is also the consultant to all the minor league affiliates of the major league club. The Chicago Cubs have affiliates in Tacoma, Washington; San Antonio, Texas; Coldwell, Idaho; Quincy, Il-

linois; and a winter league camp in Scottsdale, Arizona. These teams have a total compliment of 140 players and coaches.

The medical staff consists of a trainer with each team, the team physician and a panel of consultants in all the specialties. In addition to their interest in sports medicine and professional competence, this team must have a close rapport with the players and administrative staff.

This year professional baseball celebrated its 100th anniversary and during this period it has had sufficient time to develop certain distinctive features. Of interest to the physician is the baseball dialect. Many players have attended college and some are enrolled in graduate schools. However, when they report to the minor leagues they seem to acquire the traditional expressions used in their daily communications. By the time they have developed their athletic skills and join the major league team they have an extensive anatomic vocabulary which can be thoroughly confusing to the uninitiated. The stomach becomes the boiler, the throwing arm the hose, the eyes lamps, the legs wheels, the malingerer a jaker, the player who is a bit odd is flakey and the player who always has adhesive tape showing is referred to as a Johnson and Johnson. When a player is undressed he has had a hummer (fast ball) thrown at the middle button of his uniform shirt by the pitcher. The team physician rapidly acquires a facility for this dialect and utilizes it in establishing rapport with the players.

In the recent expansion of the major leagues the new teams paid 10 million dollars each for the personnel they obtained from the other teams. This is indicative of the relative monetary value of the professional talent. The team physician is therefore expected to provide the facilities and services required to practice preventative medicine. This is accomplished by having all new players undergo a complete *physical examination, blood counts and urinalysis during spring training in Scottsdale, Arizona. At the completion of the regular season all major league personnel have a complete physical examination, blood counts, urinalysis and chest X-ray. Where pertinent such information is communicated to their personal physician.*

In order to illustrate the variety of medical problems encountered in professional baseball players, coaches, manager and umpires, I have listed below some of the disorders seen by our staff in the past seven years.

I. Central Nervous System

  A. Concussion
  B. Convulsive Disorders
    1. Post-Traumatic
    2. Etiology undetermined

II. Endocrine and Metabolic

  A. Diabetes Mellitus
  B. Gout
  C. Rheumatoid Arthritis
  D. Heat Exhaustion

III. Infectious

  A. Bacterial
    1. Streptococcal Pharyngitis
    2. Otitis Media
    3. Otitis Externa
  B. Viral
    1. Pharyngitis—presumably viral
    2. Infectious Mononucleosis
    3. Gastro-enteritis
    4. Mumps Parotitis
    5. Mumps Pancreatitis without Parotitis
    6. Infectious Hepatitis
  C. Fungus
    1. Dermatophytosis
    2. Tinea Cruris
  D. Parasites
    1. Amebiasis
  E. Unclassified
    1. Reiter's Syndrome
    2. Prostatis

3. Urethritis

IV. Neoplasms
  A. Mixed Tumors of Parotid
  B. Lipomata
  C. Basal Cell Carcinoma

V. Cardiovascular
  A. Aortic Stenosis
  B. Coronary Insufficiency
  C. Paroxysmal Atrial Tachycandia

VI. Collagen Diseases
  A. Vasculitis

VII. Gastrointestinal Disorders
  A. Gastro-intestinal Hemorrhage due to
     duodenal ulcer
  B. Hiatal hernia

VIII. Occular Problems
  A. Astigmatism
  B. Color-Blindness

IX. Surgical Entities
  A. Acute Appendicitis
  B. Foreign Bodies
  C. Lacerations
  D. Fracture of Zygomatic Arch
  E. Fracture of Mandible

X. Psychiatric
  A. Anxiety Reaction—usually associated
     with injury
  B. Depressive Reaction

XI. Hematologic
  A. Sickle Cell Trait
  B. Myclogenous Leukemia

XII. Dental
  A. Dental Abcesses
  B. Ulceromembranous Stomatis

XIII. Non-Orthopedic Injuries
  A. Traumatic Epididymitis
  B. Scrotal Hematoma

XIV. Drug Reactions

A. Exfolliative Dermatitis

Central Nervous System Disorders

The wearing of reinforced plastic helmits has decreased the incidence of serious head injury. However, from time to time players will sustain a concussion either from a pitched ball or collision. It is our policy to hospitalize all players who have had an episode of unconsciousness or demonstrate a period of confusion following head trauma. The player is hospitalized for at least 48 hours and kept out of the line-up for another 24 hours or longer as dictated by the clinical findings. It is important to emphasize that maximal cerebral edema occurs at 48 hours and premature return to activity will expose the player to further injury at the plate if there are minor transient changes in reflex action, depth perception or diplopia.

Most all baseball players have participated in contact sports in high school and/or college. We have seen some players who have a convulsive disorder either from previous head injuries or of undetermined etiology. This is an especially difficult problem since the occurrance of seizures is not predictable, especially the petit-mal type with its transient confusional state. The consequences of such an episode occurring during batting or pitching are obvious. Control of the frequency and intensity of seizure activity can usually be achieved with appropriate therapy. Failure to achieve such control is sufficient reason to recommend discontinuing baseball as a career.

Endocrine and Metabolic Disturbances

The most challenging metabolic disorder in the young athlete is diabetes mellitus. It is apparent that diabetics who can successfully play high school baseball are not very brittle. Consequently, the diabetic in professional baseball represents a small fraction of juvenile diabetics who are relatively easily controlled with insulin and diets. These diabetics require special instruction and dietary manipulation because of the varying intensity of physical activity in extremes of environment, the altered meal schedules due to night games and travel. Several years ago we studied the activity pattern of the various positions on the team. Pedometers were utilized on selected personnel and our results would indicate that the range of distance covered by a player is 4-8 miles from the time he leaves the clubhouse for pregame workouts to his return after the game. A majority of this distance is covered while running or jogging and is influenced by the location of the dugout, his position and the number of total bases he has in a game. It is therefore obvious that control of diabetes in any professional baseball player should be highly individualized and insulin reactions are to be avoided.

Gout is a rather infrequent finding in professional baseball players. Our experience has been that if it occurs it will do so in older players, especially pitchers and will aggravate a pre-existing calcific tendonitis. Rheumatoid arthritis when it occurs in young players carries a poor career prognosis and most often is characterized by spondylitis.

We have not had any difficulty with the heat exhaustion syndrome. During a nine inning game in a hot humid stadium players will lose 5 to 8 pounds of weight. The failure to develop the heat exhaustion syndrome we feel is due to two factors. The first is that the syndrome is a failure of adaptation to environment and as such occurs early in training in a hot humid environment. Our spring training is conducted in Arizona in a low humidity environment and at the start of the season the players are fairly well heat-adapted. Secondly, during periods of high heat stress during the season all regular players take two salt tablets at the end of each inning. Some players require additional amounts of salt depending on their weight. In the past decade we have had only occasional cases of heat exhaustion and no heat stroke.

Infectious Diseases

Our most common bacterial infections have been streptococcal pharyngitis presumably contracted from children at home and otitis media and externa. Ear infections pose a real problem since all teams travel by air. We do not allow players to fly when there is an acute ear infection.

Viral infections are commonly those involving the respiratory tract and limit the player's physical capacity if swelling and obstruction of the upper passages lead to mouth breathing. Infectious mononucleosis with splenomegaly is of special concern if it occurs in an infielder or catcher who has greater occasion for body contact.

Psychiatric Problems

We have not observed any overt psychoses in our treatment of the professional athlete. However, the athlete places a rather high value on physical fitness and any injury which threatens his career and livelihood gives rise to numerous anxieties which are manifested in a number of ways. The recognition of the anxieties requires excellent confidential rapport with the player. Treatment of the injury and supportive psychotherapy are often all that is required to get the player back into the line-up in a reasonable period of time.

There has recently been a great deal of discussion in the lay press about the doping of high school, college, olympic and professional athletes. Doping consists of the use of any chemical substances not normally present in the body and not essential to a healthy person competing in athletics. The most commonly used classes of drugs appear to be analgesics, ergogenics and tranquilizers. There is evidence that amphetamines can drive trained athletes to increased performance in situations that involve sustained effort. They are not a source of additional mental or physical prowess and often lead to dangerous fatigue and therefore potential injury. Furthermore, in some individuals these drugs have dependence-producing characteristics and can lead to serious clinical and personal problems. With the protracted travel schedules and rare "off days" there is a great temptation for professional baseball players to resort to amphetamines. The almost universal availability of these drugs does little to minimize this problem. Our medical staff recognizes that there are definite medical indications for the use of amphetamines. Fortunately, we have not encountered any of these indications while treating members of our team. We therefore discourage the use of any medications by players unless they are prescribed by the medical staff.

The team physician is in charge and bears the primary and overall responsibility for maintaining the team roster and 25 healthy players. In doing this, he must be capable of making an accurate assessment of the length of disability in any illness or injury. This is dictated by the disability rules in baseball. If a player is ill or injured he cannot be replaced unless he is placed on the disability list for twenty-one days. During this period he cannot suit-up or occupy a seat in the dugout. For lesser periods of disability the player may remain on the roster but his participation will obviously be limited. In most cases the decision is fairly simple but on occasion especially with musculoskeletal injuries it is difficult to precisely define the period of disability. The decision is further complicated by the numerous pressures to get a highly skilled regular player back in the line-up. Therefore, the team physician must resist these pressures and temptations and base his conclusions on the clinical findings and his experience with similar injuries or illnesses.

Summary

The team physician has an opportunity to work with a young, exceedingly talented, highly superstitious group of athletes. He must be constantly aware of the individual variations in motivation, response to injury and training habits of the players. He is often the only non-roster member of the team who is privy to the physical or emotional problems of the moment and as such must respect the confidence and have the trust of his patients. However, he is required to inform the management of serious problems and provide the news media with a valid reason for a player's absence from the line-up. This apparent paradox is best resolved by maintaining informal lines of communication with all the responsible individuals and limiting discussions to those health problems that relate to a player's ability to perform.

Trainer's Role in High School Athletics

JOSEPH N. ABRAHAM

A RESEARCH PROJECT discloses that (1) 90 per cent of the coaches in New York State feel that first aid and caring for injuries is part of their duties, and (2) that there are few high school athletic trainers in New York State. In my opinion the regulations of the State education department prevent any individual, such as an athletic trainer, from performing certain basic duties.

What can we do about this situation? Is there a need for such an individual? What would be his duties and responsibilities? Under what supervision would he be? Would he be given a free hand or do as we do now, staying within regulations at the expense medically of the individual athletes?

Let me digress just a moment to quote from past president of the A.M.A. James E. Appel, M.D. He is also the team physician and director of health services at Franklin and Marshall College in Lancaster, Pennsylvania.

In many areas athletic directors, coaches and trainers are also giving increased emphasis to preventive and predictive medicine. This is fortunate because in no other sphere of medical interest must the physician and the public depend so heavily on the skills and judgement of nonmedical leadership.

The most learned and dedicated coach by himself, however, does not constitute quality

Presented at the Second Annual Symposium on the Medical Aspects of Sports, February 8, 1969, sponsored by the Medical Society of the State of New York.

supervision of the health needs of the athlete. He needs help . . . help from assistants who can be responsible for first aid care and emergency procedures . . . help from medical and health personnel. The decision to offer a sports program should hinge on the availability of this help.

While this help is needed at all school and adult levels of both organized and unsupervised sports activities, it is almost paradoxical that it is weakest where it is needed most: at the school level. At the college level staffs of team physicians, coaches, trainers, and health departments are usually conscientious about physical conditioning and proscribing competition by unprepared or injured athletes. But at the upper-grade and high-school levels, the community physician and his medical society can do the most to protect the least protected at the age when it is most important.

Take a look at the situation from a parent's viewpoint. He is justly proud and pleased, like most parents, when he learns that his son has made the squad. But if the boy is seriously injured while carrying out an assignment that he is not able to handle because of some minor or temporary disability, the outlook is considerably changed. Not only is the parent faced with the burden of medical expense but with a much more important worry, his son's condition.

School officials have a perfect right to feel that the school is performing a real service for both the boy and the parent by sponsoring an organized athletic program. Equally, parents have the right to assume that the school should be responsible for the physical condition of athletes who perform for the school in contests for which admission is charged. Admittedly, there are two sides to the question.

The coach is in the most difficult spot of all. Most coaches have studied first aid and treatment for minor injuries. But any coach supervising a large squad actually does not have the time to do a real trainer's job. Another problem faced by every coach is presented by the boy who is so anxious to play that he intentionally does not mention the slight bruise or sprain he has incurred. The sad ending to this story is that the boy, in favoring the minor injury, usually leaves himself wide open in a more vulnerable spot. Thus, he winds up with a more serious injury.

James A. Nicholas, M.D., an orthopedic surgeon, has strong interest in sports medicine. He is the team physician and orthopedic consultant to the New York Jets and orthopedic consultant to West Point Military Academy and a number of high schools in the New York City area. He declares that the biggest difference between college and high school is that the high school player who is hurt is not given an immediate examination unless he is badly hurt. If the boy receives a sprain, it may be ignored because it was not severe enough. Or he may go home before it swells. No one knows of the injury because the boy has not told anyone about it. This leaves him subject to another more severe injury. Here then is the big difference: in college, athletic injuries are taken care of by a specific person. In the secondary level, there is a question as to who will take care of the injuries.

There are, approximately, 750 secondary schools in New York State participating in athletics in one form or another. I sent a questionnaire to the high schools in New York State listed in the high schools coaches' directory. It was as short and simple as possible to encourage replies. The response was excellent: 453 schools reported, 61 per cent of the total (Fig. 1).

Interpretation of questionnaire

Twenty per cent of these schools do not require a record of the boy's medical history.

It is a foregone conclusion that the boy's medical history is a necessity. Physical examinations are given by most schools before participation is allowed. The time that physicians are most frequently available in the area of play is at varsity football games when they are present 68 per cent of the time. In all other sports, the percentage runs much lower than this. For example, in basketball, out of 422 schools, only 14.3 per cent report a physician in the area. In junior varsity game football, the percentage is 35.8 In freshman football, the percentage is 31.6. In practice sessions physicians are present for only 8 per cent in those schools replying to the questionnaire. Percentages are low for all other sports. Except for the coach, for 62.5 per cent of the time there is no specific individual responsible for injury when the physician is not on the field.

The duties of the coach, other than coaching, in over 85 per cent of the replies are (1) collection and issue of equipment, (2) supervision of locker room, (3) seeing that the injured player is taken to the physician or hospital, (4) checking all minor injuries and treating for first aid (5) applying all protection taping for practice and games, and (6) in 50 per cent of the replies for maintenance of equipment.

The heart of our problem lies in the fact that the coaches are burdened with too much responsibility. They may be able to handle adequately all of the other duties listed, and if these are not done immediately, no harm is done, with the exception of getting the

FIGURE 1. The questionnaire and responses.

Do you require a past record of a boy's medical history? Yes—363
No— 62
No Answer— 28

Please check:

	Physical Exam	Physician at Area	Per cent	Vehicle on Field or Area	Stretcher on Field or Area	First Aid Kit on Area	Per cent
Vr football game	354	305	67.3	244	334	368	81.2
JV football game	326	192	35.8	147	299	336	74.2
Fr football game	235	143	31.6	97	212	242	45.4
Basketball Vr & JV	422	65	14.3	95	245	413	91.2
Wrestling Vr & JV	275	54	11.9	62	186	279	61.5
Baseball Vr	406	39	8.6	90	196	396	87.4
Lacrosse Vr	62	10	2.2	20	39	68	98.0
Practice session football	310	37	8.1	79	214	326	71.9

If a doctor is not available, is there a specific individual on the field or play area responsible for injuries *other than the coach* to give first aid?

Yes	133	29.4%
No	283	62.5%
No answer	37	8.1%

FIGURE I. *continued*

Please check the following *if the Coach* is responsible for the following:
(If anyone other than the Coach is responsible, check "No").

	Yes	Per cent	No	No Answer
Ordering of equipment	227	50.0	215	11
Collect and issue equipment	389	85.9	58	6
Maintenance of equipment	263	58.1	181	9
Maintenance of field	86	18.9	346	21
Supervision of locker room and school	393	86.6	53	7
Sign vouchers	143	31.6	295	15
Scheduling	160	35.3	279	14
Cancellations	173	38.2	269	11
Officials	145	32.0	298	10
Budget	135	29.8	306	12
Transportation of athletes in returning home	148	32.7	292	13
Seeing that the injured player is taken to the doctor's or to the hospital	397	87.6	69	5
Check all minor injuries and treat for first aid	403	88.9	40	10
Check all insurance records	124	27.4	312	17
Apply all protection taping for practice and games	406	89.6	44	3

Playing Conditions and Equipment
To what degree would you attribute player injuries to poor field conditions?

Never	69	15.2%
Sometimes	304	67.1%
Frequently	58	12.8%
Very frequently	13	2.9%
No answer	9	2.0%

Do you have a first aid room available for injured players?

Yes	218	48.2%
No	229	50.5%
No answer	6	1.3%

Do you require a tetanus shot within two years of participation?

Yes	112	24.0%
No	313	69.0%
No answer	28	7.0%

In your opinion, do you consider the equipment available to you a source of injuries, such as poorly fitted equipment, or equipment not good enough to protect the players?

Yes	25	5.5%
No	419	92.5%
No answer	9	2.0%

In your opinion, do you consider the range of ages as a detriment to some players?

Yes	153	33.8%
No	289	63.8%
No answer	11	2.4%

Along this same line does the schedule of one team in a higher class participating against a lower league offer a higher incidence of injuries?

Yes	166	33.6%
No	244	
No answer	43	

Are records kept for all injured players?

Yes	422	93%
No	27	
No answer	4	

When a transfer registers and participates is there a medical record of his past?

Yes	328	72%
No	91	
No answer	34	

Procedure for Injured on Field
After initial first aid, is there any formal procedure followed regardless of the nature of the injury?

Yes	348	76%
No	86	
No answer	19	

Who is responsible for follow-up of injury?

Coach	277	61.1%
Nurse	223	49.0%
Doctor	142	31.3%
Other	96	

player to the hospital, giving first aid, and applying protection tape. Many teams have only one person as coach and, if lucky, two. All of these duties cannot be handled by coaches if they are to do a good job, and of the replies returned, 88.9 per cent of the coaches feel that first aid is so much of their responsibility that they list it as one of their duties.

In addition, 82.8 per cent of the coaches attribute at least some of the injuries to poor field conditions, and 86.9 per cent indicate that the coach is responsible for this, too. In 48.2 per cent of the schools there is no first aid room available. Only 1.3 per cent gave no answer to this question.

We need no more detail from this survey to point out that most of the medical coverage is the responsibility of the coach; 85.9 per cent are expected to include this in their coaching duties. As a result medical coverage is not adequate for a large number of individuals. The coach has too many duties to perform. Taking care of any injury may not be possible as immediately as it should be.

Resources for improvement

If we have 25,000 participants with 8,000 injuries, and we can lessen the injuries by 2 per school, this would drop the percentage rates 10 to 15 per cent. Just being aware of the injury problem can reduce injuries. Where clinics have been held, injuries dropped 10 to 20 per cent. For this purpose information can be obtained from two organizations in New York State which keep statistics of injuries in the high school program: the New York State High School Athletic Protection Plan, Inc., and the New York State Public High School Athletic Association, which has dealt mainly with football injuries, more injuries occurring here than in any other sport. "Dutch" Hafner has at his disposal a book of vital statistics to help anyone who wants information to help prevent injuries.* My charts indicate in what areas injuries occur, so that all persons associated with leading the sport may know what to expect. Better yet, if a specific individual is assigned to a team with sole medical responsibility, injuries can be cut from 10 to 40 per cent.

*New York State Department of Education, New York State Athletic Association, Albany, New York.

Injuries in some areas occur only 10 per cent of the time, in some areas 30 to 50 per cent of the time. I repeat, it has been found that where there have been clinics and schools to enable coaches to understand and be aware of injuries, the percentages have dropped.

No answer is foolproof, but, with this knowledge, all phases of the athletic program can begin a program to offer proper medical care for safe participation in sports, including the presence of a physician as often as possible for games and practice sessions. If this is not possible, a second coach or responsible person should be in charge to handle the injury phase of athletics.

S. E. Bilik, M.D.,† says that he has adhered to the principle that methods we use in medicine and in training have a thoroughly sound psychological basis. When you have a man who has the basic logic and coolness under fire to recognize the immediate problem adequately and who adheres to sound scientific routine of treatment, you have the ideal man for the profession.

Athletic trainer

Let us call our responsible person an athletic trainer. He should be qualified to give service in the following areas: (1) in athletics the primary concern of the trainer is management and prevention of athletic injuries. Most athletic injuries are accidents. Under the guidance of the medical profession, the athletic trainer must strive to prevent these accidents. He can do this through daily supervision of safety factors on all athletic fields, eliminating all undue hazards, issuing equipment with care, and supervising all training menus. Because of the brief time element involved in athletics, and the inability to rehabilitate injured athletes completely in season, the athletic trainer must be skilled in preventive and supportive strappings. The athletic trainer, in the management of athletic injuries, must give "on the field first aid" and follow up and carry out in detail the physician's prescription for continued care and rehabilitation. (2) In physical education the athletic trainer should assume the responsibility for the care of all injuries in both physical edu-

†Speech presented at 12th Annual Meeting Eastern Athletic Trainers Association, January 17, 1961, New York, New York.

cation and intramural sports. There is a great similarity between these injuries and those of interschool athletics. Therefore, there is sound justification for the listing of all injuries in physical education, athletics, and intramural sports under the term "athletic injury."

Besides being members of an athletic medical team, trainers are in the unique position of being closely associated with coaches, players, and administrators. Athletic trainers should coordinate, under medical supervision and, with the cooperation of administrators and coaches, the total program of training and conditioning for as long as the athlete is the responsibility of the athletic department. This should be a four-phase responsibility: prevention of injuries, first aid, follow-up treatment, and rehabilitation.

According to the best sources available, the National Athletic Trainer Association program was designed to encourage the nation's high schools to seek qualified men as trainers. The program includes major study in physical education and necessary courses required by the states for a teaching license. Also included in the degree program is a total of twenty-four semester hours in physical, biologic, and social sciences. Three objectives have been fulfilled by the program: (1) a curriculum which would give the individual the broadest teaching certificate possible, (2) a curriculum which would have prephysical therapy courses accepted by an American Medical Association-approved physical therapy school, and (3) a curriculum that will prepare men in the management and the prevention of athletic injuries.

There are many trainers who, if given the same educational background as physical therapists, would use a more standard method of applying technics. There should be emphasis on the need for proper training in physical therapy modalities. Many of the training rooms average 4,000 to 4,500 treatments each school year. That is proof of the need for adequate training in indications and contraindications that at present can only be taught in physical therapy schools.

The formulation of this program was intended solely to create guidelines and standards of education for colleges and universities to follow in preparing the future athletic trainer for the secondary school level. The program was adopted in June, 1959, by the National Athletic Trainer's Association and was meant to encourage more qualified athletic training. The Association, in its hope to raise standards of the profession, will continually seek to increase educational qualifications on all levels.

To repeat for emphasis, there is a need for personnel to help prevent injuries and follow standing orders of a physician when he may not be present or available.

Physical therapists should be able to participate in this program, but I regret to say that a survey of New York State physical therapy schools shows the number of senior men graduating in 1967 pursuing a degree or certificate in physical therapy was only 22. In the whole State of New York, we had 22 men graduating from physical therapy schools. Will they be able to handle the number of injured high school players alone?

Comment

We should take a hard look at the number of persons injured. Who is available to take care of them and their injuries? The physician is much too busy to attend practice sessions and games. If physical therapists are not available, then who should be appointed to be present at every practice and game? Who should see that a physician is called when necessary, or see that the injured player is taken to the physician's office or hospital or home, or told not to practice until he has been seen by a physician.

So that the word trainer will be understood by everyone, it is my contention that this person be so designated by the school. He may be called an assistant coach, first aid man, or other terminology. However, so that we all understand one another, I use the term trainer. He will be the individual to whom all injuries will be reported immediately, and he will see that the proper care is taken of these injuries by the proper people with follow-up of these injuries.

The State of New York should set up the following duties for a trainer:

1. He should work under the direct supervision of a physician in all matters pertaining to the health and medical care of individuals actively engaged in the college and high school athletic program.

2. He should be responsible for the training room.

3. He should keep written records of all injuries.

4. He should be on duty throughout the day and be on call when needed.

5. He should attend all games and practices.

6. He should render first aid in case of injury, for example the strap bandage, and apply protective equipment.

7. He should refer all injury cases to a physician.

8. He should assist the physician in the examination of athletes, record all results, list old injuries, and keep a permanent file.

9. He should operate therapeutic equipment on orders of the physician.

10. He should maintain high standards of training procedure correlated with the educational policy of the school.

11. He should record and check supplies requisition needs.

12. He should be loyal to, and cooperate with, the coaching personnel, physician, and authority in terms of total service to the team.

We have seen from the cold hard facts that (1) many injuries occur on the secondary level; (2) many injuries may be prevented; (3) a physician is not available most of the time; and (4) 88.9 per cent of the coaches have indicated they feel that injuries are their responsibility along with collection and issue of equipment, supervision of locker rooms, and maintenance of equipment.

Conclusion

If a responsible person were delegated to take care of these duties or the injury phase itself, it is certain that the percentage of injuries would drop by a large percentage. If secondary schools would appoint this responsible person, they could save more than the amount of his salary through lower insurance premiums. This has been proved by schools here in New York State. The state is leaning toward certifying coaching sports. This is good, for certain qualifications would have to be met.

I'm sure when people realize the problem they will try to solve it.

I may have painted a dark picture, but it is easily seen. With the help of the medical profession, schools can be made to realize that there is one more step. It is education, training, and appointment of a responsible person to more nearly approach our goal: complete safety in athletics.

Sports Medicine in Urban New York

DANIEL H. MANFREDI, M.D., F.A.C.S.

Sports injuries in a large metropolitan city like New York comprise almost every known type of athletic trauma, ranging from injuries sustained in a little municipal park ski slope or ice rink to the ones suffered in the indoor and outdoor big-time sports events. Many of these contests have present at the sports arena medical personnel who can render first aid or definitive treatment to the injured athlete. Many others do not have medical supervision in attendance so that hospital emergency rooms are frequently swamped with injured sand-lot or medically unsupervised athletes.

The majority of our city universities, high schools, and professional teams have physicians present at all their games. On the other hand, there are a great many sports events that lack proper medical supervision during play. Some of these athletic groups have adopted the trainer supervision method in which the trainer will call a physician if he deems it necessary. Many of these trainers nowadays are well-qualified persons with an adequate first aid training and are capable of handling an emergency while awaiting medical help. The old image of a trainer being a short, fat, cigar-smoking, tough guy, wearing a dirty sweat shirt and carrying a bucket of water and a towel in his hand, has long since disappeared. This trainer-present situation is the next best thing to having a physician in attendance.

The advantages of having a physician immediately available at an athletic event are numerous and incalculable. Athletes feel more reassured and at ease knowing that a physician is available in case of accidental injury. They play with more confidence and efficiency when they know that proper medical emergency treatment will be rendered immediately. The agonizing and stressful waiting period before help arrives is eliminated.

Many coaches and trainers are happy to have a physician present who can render decisions as to the playability of a player. This relieves them of a serious responsibility. The question frequently arises, "What qualifications should a team physician possess?" Since his duties encompass the treatment of trauma to the abdomen, chest, bones, joints, soft tissues, head, neck, skin, and so on, he must be a medically versatile healer. He must also have an interest and knowledge of athletes and their sports. He should also share in an undemonstrative manner in the victories and defeats of his cared-for athletes. Any graduate physician can be a team's physician, provided he has had the proper training and has an open mind to call in the help of a specialist when needed. The ideal team physician should be a general surgeon with training in trauma of soft tissues, bone, and viscera, coupled with a medical school knowledge of medicine, psychiatry, orthopedics, and pediatrics. He must also be very sympathetic and have understanding and patience to listen to all the various and sundry aches, pains, and complaints that anxious athletes consciously and subconsciously develop. If the physician has all these attributes, with time he will gradually develop an avid interest in the sport, become mildly addicted, and will find himself exercising great self-restraint in preventing himself from advising the coach as to proper strategy in play. After a long term of office, a team physician will find himself gradually sliding into the aforementioned pattern.

The playing arena can be compared to an oversized experimental laboratory in trauma where the experimental animals are the athletes. Here, under direct observation of the physician, the causes, mechanics, physiology, and treatment of injuries can be accurately analyzed. The team physician therefore becomes a trauma researcher with data being presented to him throughout a contest. He may come to certain definite conclusions concerning various traumatic conditions. A case in point would be the occurrence last year of two simultaneous tears of the Achilles tendon in track athletes on a cold day when insufficient warming-up time was allowed before full sprinting. He may suspect a tendinitis occurring in a pitcher's shoulder following a particular type of thrown curved ball. A tennis elbow may occur when using a racket with a certain motion. A knee injury may occur following a type of tackle, or a boxing injury may result from an improperly placed punch.

Are sports injuries different from trauma sustained in nonathletic events? Not exactly, when they are analyzed anatomically. Anyone can trip and sprain an ankle, fracture a wrist, or injure a knee cartilage without playing football. A rupture of the spleen or abdominal viscera does not require a head-on football tackle as its cause. While we do find certain types of injuries more prevalent in athletes than nonathletes, we can reason that exposure to contact, or more correctly, collision, is more frequent in sports events.

Most organized athletic teams require pretraining physical examinations to rule out any diseases, deformities, or predisposing factors to injuries. The procedure has helped to keep the casualty records at a very low level.

The immediate care of an injured athlete is of utmost importance and can prevent catastrophes or future complications. Splinting where the patients lie, use of stretchers, control of bleeding, ice packs to soft-tissue and joint injuries, nonambulation of suspected fracture patients,

fasting for patients with suspected visceral injuries, maintaining airways, and proper handling of cervical and back vertebral injuries, are some of the basic principles to be observed on the playing field.

Types of injuries

Specific injuries for certain sports follow a pattern of physical activity. A tennis player on serving a ball may rise on his toes sustaining a tear of his plantaris tendon. This form of trauma has a typical diagnostic history. The player complains of sudden sharp pain in his calf, looks around to see if he was hit by a ball or pellet, and is sure that he heard a loud sound as the tendon ruptured. It is very disabling, and strapping and a heel lift shorten the two to four weeks of convalescence. A baseball pitcher complains of pains in the anterior shoulder after a fast-pitched curved ball. Clinical tests may reveal tenderness over the short head of the biceps muscle with certain motions aggravating the pains. A tendinitis diagnosis is suspected. He is helped by hydrocortisone injections and exercises. A football player may complain of pains in the knee over the medial portion with locking and swelling of the joint. Examination reveals tenderness over the medial cartilage of the knee joint. Here a possible torn cartilage is diagnosed, and an operation is scheduled. Ankle injuries occur in all sports and may vary from ligamentous tears and chip fractures to tibial and fibular fractures with varying separations. The treatments will vary from adhesive strappings to casts and open operations.

Injuries of the knee rank as the number one trauma of football. A hard side tackle by a 200-pound opponent to a runner's knee whose football cleats have anchored his leg produces a sequence of traumatic results. The medial cartilage is the first to go, followed in turn by the lateral collateral ligament, and finally the cruciate ligaments. These injuries, when severe enough, will require surgical intervention. Dislocations of the knee do occur at times and are considered enormous emergencies since the blood supply to the leg may be impaired. Soccer players, despite their protective shin guards, are frequent victims of spiking to their lower extremities. Dislocations do occur in rare situations. Scrotal injuries due to trauma produce great shock and require ice packs, elevation, sedatives, and rest. Intra-abdominal injuries to viscera have become more frequent because of the head-spearing type of tackling that is presently being practiced. These injuries require careful observation and decisions not to allow continuation of play until it has been ascertained that no intra-abdominal viscera are ruptured. Coaches and players will frequently plead for return to action, and a serious catastrophe may result. I recall one football player who sustained a ruptured duodenum and who pleaded with me to permit him back into the game since it was only his wind that had been knocked out.

In the upper extremities we find that fingers are frequently dislocated in baseball and football players, and early reduction on the spot is good therapy. Wrists may be sprained or fractured, and here again early reduction and immobilization are indicated. Elbows can be dislocated or fractured with severe ligamentous tears. Early x-ray studies should be performed to rule out fractures and intra-articular fragments of bone that have wandered into the joint. A common elbow injury is the so-called "tennis elbow." It is a painful affliction of the outer aspect of the joint with inability to grasp well or raise medium-weight objects. It is not confined wholly to tennis players, since golfers, baseball pitchers, violinists, typists, dentists, and even proctologists can be victims of this crippling entity. Treatment with injections of cortisone plus exercise and sedation help to alleviate the suffering.

The shoulder dislocates more frequently than any other joint in competitive sports. Early attempts at reduction before muscle spasm sets in are usually successful. No immediate participation following this injury is permitted. The shoulder is a common site for tendinitis in baseball pitchers. It is aggravated by constant rotation of the humeral head under the short head of the biceps tendon which irritates the undersurface. These cases are also treated by injections of cortisone and strengthening exercises. Bursitis and cuff injuries are another cause of painful shoulder which plague many baseball pitchers.

The head receives many blows in collision sports with varying grades of concussion and occasional fractures. The use of stretchers to remove players from the playing field may prevent serious internal cerebral hemorrhage. Fractures about the face have diminished because of the protective gear now worn. Nasal fractures with displacement should be moulded between thumbs on the spot and held in position by splints.

Neck injuries including so-called whiplash and cervical disk abnormal conditions are associated with neuritides of the spinal nerves and can be very disabling. There is constant talk about prohibiting boys with long thin necks from playing football because of their susceptibility to easy injury of the neck.

Fractures of the clavicles are common and are treated by the conventional methods. Back injuries can be disabling and require patience and accurate diagnosis for their treatment. Fractures of all the long bones may occur in all sports, and early splinting is the basic emergency treatment.

This thumbnail sketch is a brief analysis of the injuries I have seen during my twenty years with athletic teams.

Conclusion

In conclusion, it must appear obvious that treatment of injuries in athletes is no different from treatment of trauma in nonathletes. The advantages of being at the scene of the accident and observing its mechanics is twofold. The physician can evaluate the abnormal condition before spasm and further injury are sustained. The treatment can be initiated immediately and can be of emergency nature of definitive as described previously.

The question often arises, why are certain traumatic conditions occurring so constantly in sports contests. The answer is naturally because of the greater exposure of the athlete to collision and violence. If we could define war in medical terms as an epidemic of trauma, then sports injuries could be classified as mild endemic outbreaks of traumatic disease. When these sporadic outbreaks occur with regularity in specified areas, they require investigation. The cause may be poor coaching, poor equipment, inadequate medical supervision, poor officiating, or improper health habits.

At present there is a beehive of activity in the preventive traumatology studies being conducted by numerous organized committees of sports medicine. Coaches, trainers, university officials, parents, physicians, and the public are all eager to see the injury factor removed from the sports arena. That goal is slowly being achieved.

The great physical and mental benefits that sports provide to our youth are incontestable. Sports build the sound bodies which in turn nurture the sound mind. As physicians associated with the sports program of our youth, we must help to promulgate this ancient Greek doctrine.

Nutrition in Athletes

NUTRITION IN SPORT

By J. G. P. WILLIAMS, M.B., F.R.C.S.Ed., D.Phys.Med.

The importance of nutrition for health has long been recognized and it is well known that the Greek Olympic athletes in the ancient world took very great care over their diets. Indeed, so diet conscious did the early Olympians become that they came to present a singularly unathletic picture and, as Plato stated, 'are liable to most dangerous illnesses if they depart in ever so slight a degree from their customary regimen'.

From time immemorial it would seem that various particular foodstuffs have had attributed to them invigorating properties, at times amounting almost to the miraculous. Among cannibals the devouring of certain selected parts of one's enemy's anatomy (for example the heart) was regarded as conducive to development of great strength and courage. So assiduous has the cult of certain foodstuffs been throughout the ages, even up to the excessive use of wheat germ oil at the present time, that it has been difficult to determine where to define the borderline between nutrition and doping. It is interesting to note in this latter context that the role of pure glucose has come in for the attention of those seeking to legislate against dope in sport (Williams 1968).

It is therefore hardly surprising that the whole question of nutrition in sport is bedevilled with fads, fancies and old wives' tales, and more and more weird and wonderful diets are constantly being put forward on the basis that they have particular qualities in providing just what the athlete needs.

BASIC FACTS

From a practical point of view, the whole question of sports nutrition is perfectly straightforward and involves little if any mystique. In essence, the sportsman, like anybody else, requires adequate amounts of the three basic foodstuffs: carbohydrate, protein and fat. These basic foodstuffs are usually presented in the proportion of protein—1, fat—1, carbohydrate—4, although where the higher-calorie diets are concerned it is usual to reduce slightly the proportion of carbohydrate.

The introduction to the section on the 'Principles of dietetics' in the 9th edition of 'Samson Wright's Applied Physiology' presents as succinct a summary of dietetic principles as any;

An adequate diet must have a caloric value sufficient to provide for the requirements of basal metabolism . . . and the needs of varying degrees of muscular work. It must have adequate amounts of protein (essential amino-acids), fat, carbohydrate, water and salts (ions) in suitable proportions and an ample vitamin content'. (Keele and Neil, 1961).

This principle, of course, holds true for the diet of sportsmen.

In general, by virtue of his high energy expenditure, the sportsman will require a greater caloric intake than the average person. In most Western European communities the eating habits and customs are such that the vast majority of the population obtain their basic foodstuffs in roughly the correct proportions and in a satisfactory form. Whereas the normal daily caloric requirement for the average worker will be of the order of 2,700 to 3000 calories, the sportsman undergoing severe training may require half as much again, or more, with a total dietary need of up to 5000 calories a day (Ruffell, 1962). These food requirements are usually provided quite simply by increasing all round the food intake without in any way significantly altering the proportions of the different constituents of the diet.

Because of the quantities involved, however, it may be that the sportsman finds an all-round increase in food intake to some degree indigestible, and many will therefore cut down on bread and potatoes, preferring to increase proportionately their intake of meat, cheese, fruit and green vegetables. Unfortunately, this type of dietary modification may involve considerable expense and it is not uncommon to find some of the financially less well endowed sportsmen making up their caloric requirements with large amounts of carbohydrate (bread, potatoes, cereals).

PALATABILITY

The whole question of total food intake is related not only to expense but to palatability. It is, of course, axiomatic that many of the more tasty foods are more expensive. Unfortunately, either because of the fact that the expensive foods are themselves attractive or because legend endows them with particular qualities (Robson and Herron, 1959), many sportsmen will deprive themselves to an unnecessary extent in other directions in order to obtain these foods. (The food value in a pound of fillet steak is hardly significantly greater than in an equivalent weight of meat taken from one of the less attractive cuts.) Because, however, the sportsman has to take food in large quantities, it is essential for this food to be as interesting and palatable as possible, and it is only when the less expensive items are prepared with a considerable amount of care that they can measure up in attraction to the expensive delicacies.

The importance of palatability of diet cannot be overstressed. Athletic training is, at best, an uncomfortable and tedious process if the sportsman concerned is desirous of achieving a high standard of performance. During training he is constantly fighting against boredom, staleness and the attraction of other, less uncomfortable activities. It is therefore important that factors which would tend to depress the sportsman and render his whole regimen even less attractive should be eliminated so far as possible. There is no doubt that a dreary diet is a most potent cause of disaffection among sportsmen (Van Itallie et al., 1960).

Quite apart from the obvious need for appropriate amounts of the basic foodstuffs, attractively presented, the athlete's diet may require some additional supplementation in relation to vitamins. In the first place, quite a number of sportsmen will obtain at least part of their dietary intake from institutional sources: for example, college refectory, works canteen, or office restaurant. Food prepared along mass production lines is often overcooked and this leads to a loss particularly of vitamin C. Because of the importance of this vitamin in suprarenal metabolism, it is usually necessary for the athlete to supplement his diet with additional vitamin C. Here fresh fruit (whole or juice) or fruit essences (for example, 'ribena') are a valuable source of additional vitamin C and an important part of the sportsman's diet.

Vitamins of the B series seem also to be particularly required by athletes, since especially aneurine and riboflavine appear to be needed in recovery from fatigue. Vitamin E, the active principle of wheat germ oil, has been claimed to be of benefit, but there is no evidence to support this claim.

The importance of adequate mineral intake is obvious, bearing in mind that sodium chloride is lost in considerable quantities in sweating, and a daily intake of 2 grammes is the minimum. The average diet provides four times this amount, but even this is inadequate when heavy sweating and particularly heavy, unaccustomed sweating, is induced. In conditions therefore giving rise to a great deal of sweating to which the athlete is not used (for example, in a sudden heat wave) additional salt is a necessity.

In general, as I have pointed out elsewhere (Williams, 1965):

'It is reasonable to suggest that too much fuss is often made of the diet of the athlete or sportsman . . . There is little, if any, need to modify the normal (by Western European and American standards) diet other than by increasing in proportion the amounts of food as needed to meet the average requirements'.

SPECIAL DIETARY NEEDS

These comments cover the basic day-to-day needs of the sportsman in training. Special circumstances, however, do arise when a sportsman is involved in physical activities which extend over a protracted period without a break (Creff and Berard, 1966). Examples of this type of activity include marathon cycling events (for example, the Land's End to John O'Groats record), ultra-long-distance canoe races such as the Devizes to Westminster, and the Oxford to Westminster rowing record which has recently attracted the attention of a number of crews. In these events, which last over a period of several hours, the sportsman has to take in food as he goes along. When the activity is strenuous, as in the examples given above, the caloric requirement may be as high as 1000 calories an hour.

The average individual will tolerate only relatively small amounts of glucose over a period and it thus becomes necessary to provide the caloric intake in the form of suitable broths and stews which are carbohydrate based. Thus, watery rice pudding, fruit juices and oatmeal mash are examples of preparations often used. These may be supplemented by dried fruit and chocolate, but it is generally considered advisable to avoid fat in any quantity and any great amount of protein. Adequate salt must be added to the diet for long-duration events and suitable fluid intake must be provided.

WEIGHT

For most people, the range of optimum weight is largely fixed by constitutional factors. The classification of physique using the three point somatotype is already well established, and it has been shown clearly that the basic shape of an individual remains peculiar to himself, to some extent regardless of dietary variations (Williams, 1965).

When a sportsman goes into training, there is usually an initial weight loss which is due partly to the elimination of excess tissue fluids and partly to metabolism of stored fat. As training proceeds, the weight trend is reversed and the sportsman gains weight, due to an increase in muscle bulk. The extent of the increase will vary according to the basic body type.

In the case of the mesomorph, the weight gain is much greater than in the case of the ectomorph. Once a regular pattern of training is established there should follow little variation in weight, and sudden unexpected or large variations require investigation. There is, however, one exception to this basic premise and this is the case of the 'power event' competitior (for example, shot-putter, weight-lifter) whose aim is to increase body bulk to a considerable extent. In these cases the diet is often excessive and the risk to the athlete is of increasing not only the total muscle bulk but also the stored fat. Excessive fat storage is of value only to the long-distance swimmer.

In some sports, of course, weight is a disadvantage and some sportsmen may require a diet which will enable them to keep their weight below certain limits. Examples of people in this category include boxers, wrestlers, jockeys and coxswains. Provided that weight reduction is made only at the expense of stored fat, no clinical danger results. When, however, weight reduction can only be achieved either by excessive fluid loss (drying out) or frank starvation there follows some clinical risk. In such cases it is essential to provide a diet which will present to the sportsman all his needs: caloric, protein, mineral and vitamin. If on such a diet he cannot keep his weight down then it is essential that he should be persuaded to accept sports participation in a higher weight category. It would appear that a diet of 2,300 calories a day should be regarded as somewhere near the minimum for active participation in sport.

FEEDING HABITS

In addition to the obvious need for adequate intake of food, the sportsman is faced with a need to govern his feeding habits in relation to his physical activity. Comment has already been made on the importance of a palatable diet and this point cannot be over-stressed.

At the same time, it is important that meals should be presented at appropriate and suitable times (Bensley, 1951). During the period shortly after ingestion of food, blood is shunted into the visceral vessel to assist the processes of digestion. This immediately diminishes the amount of circulating blood available to supply active muscles. In consequence, if physical activity (particularly strenuous physical activity) is undertaken within an hour or two of completing a meal, either there is a fall off in the muscular circulation, which can, for example, give rise to post-prandial swimmer's cramp, or the visceral shunt is reversed, giving rise to indigestion and possible malabsorption with a possibility of diarrhœa and/or vomiting. Furthermore, if the food ingested has been of the gas-producing variety which ferments in the intestine (for example, beans, cucumber and radishes) the individual may become the victim of wind colic.

Not only is the timing of meals important, but also the presentation of the various courses. Fresh fruit juices stimulate digestive juices. Fish and meat stimulate gastric secretion; fats delay digestion. Sugars, by their osmotic effect, draw fluid from the gastric lining and so give rise to feelings of satiation.

The proportion of the diet to be accepted at the different meals is also of considerable significance to the sportsman. In general, the breakfast should be fairly substantial, but not too much so, particularly if much physical exertion is to be undertaken in the early part of the morning (Tuttle et al., 1950, 1959). Luncheon must be light and easily digested, whilst the main meal of the day should be the evening meal. This last meal should take place some time after the conclusion of the day's physical activity and at least an hour, preferably two, before the individual retires to bed.

'MAGIC FOODS'

Reference has already been made to the remarkable extent to which special properties are attributed to various foodstuffs. It seems now established that there is no evidence that the diet immediately before a short-term athletic event can be manipulated in such a way as to improve performance. Over and over again extravagant claims are made for different types of food as dietary constituents for sportsmen. Wheat germ oil has already been quoted as a case in point. What seems much more likely is that there will follow a deterioration in performance when adequate diet is not provided. From every point of view sportsmen and athletes must be discouraged from seeking a 'super food' to provide them with a substitute for hard work in training. It is not surprising that questions of nutrition have been raised in recent legislation among governing bodies in sport aimed at stamping out the practice of doping. The use of drugs and 'super foods' to enhance athletic performance must be contrary to the spirit of the sport.

SUMMARY

(1) The importance of an adequate diet for the maintenance of health in sportsmen is stressed.

182

(2) There is no special peculiarity about the sportsman's diet. Essentially the sportsman requires much the same type of diet as anyone else, but with a greater caloric intake.

(3) There is a case for including in the sportsman's diet additional vitamin C, vitamin B complex, and salt.

(4) For certain ultra-long-duration events special provision must be made to maintain caloric intake. Such provision will be based upon carbohydrate broths and stews, containing additional salt. Glucose in large quantities is not well tolerated.

(5) Whatever the form of diet taken, it is essential that it shall be palatable and attractive. Dreary food inevitably leads to disillusionment, with a consequent deleterious effect on training.

(6) Weight is a fair guide to the adequacy of the diet. A sportsman will usually lose a little weight when he starts training but the process is soon reversed. Once training is fully established, weight should remain more or less constant.

(7) Weight gain may be required for power event competitors and in these cases additional food intake is given. The risk of over-eating, with fat deposit, must be stressed.

(8) Great care must be taken in providing adequate nutrition for sportsmen who require to maintain low weight levels.

(9) Timing of food in relation to physical activity is important, and in general the main meal should be taken late in the day, after the conclusion of all heavy activity.

Although there is considerable doubt as to whether maintenance of an adequate diet can enhance performance, there is no doubt whatever that performance can be significantly impaired when a less than adequate diet is consumed. The best diet for the athlete is one which he enjoys and one which, at the same time, provides a variety of nutritious foods in amounts adequate to maintain his weight at an optimal level.

References

Bensley, E. H. (1951): ·Canad. med. Ass. J., 64, 503.

Creff, A. F., and Berard, L. (1966): 'Sport et Alimentation', La Table Ronde, Paris.

Keele, C. A., and Neil, E. (1961): 'Samson Wright's Applied Physiology', 10th ed., Oxford University Press, London.

Plato 'The Republic', Para. 2, 404.

Robson, H. E., and Herron, R. J. (1959): Phys. Educ., 11, 4.

Ruffell, J. (1962): in 'Sports Medicine', ed. by J. G. P. Williams, Edward Arnold & Sons Ltd., London.

Tuttle, W. A., Daum, K., Martin, C., and Myers, L. (1950): J. Amer. diet. Ass., 26, 332.

——, Wilson, M., and Daum, K. (1959): J. appl. Physiol., 1, 545.

Van Itallie, T. B., Sinisterra, L., and Stare, F. J. (1960): in 'Science and Medicine of Exercise and Sports', ed. by W. R. Johnson, Harper Bros., New York.

Williams, J. G. T. (1965): 'Medical Aspects of Sport and Physical Fitness', Pergamon Press, Oxford.

—— (1968): in 'Doping in Sport', Symposium, British Association of Sport Medicine, in the press.

S. J. P. TURCO, M.D.

DIETS IN ATHLETICS

Food Fads Cannot Replace a Balanced Diet for Athletic Performance

The performance of an athlete in events which test his physical functions to the utmost is largely dependent upon a ready supply of the nutrient materials required by his working tissues. The body is an extremely complex biochemical laboratory, with countless complex ingredients of specific composition and physiological function. With a sensible, intelligent diet a healthy body is ever-ready to meet the most exacting demands upon it. For intelligent planning of a diet for the training table one must have clear understanding of the physiological principle of nutrition. Many books have been written on this subject and can be obtained in most any libraries. In dietetics one must avoid fads.

FADS

False and controversial diet theories are still influencing the training table diets of many high schools and colleges. Too many good foods high in nutritional value are banned for no sound physiological or nutritional reasons, such as milk, pork, candy, pie, and cake. If these items are eaten as part of the well-balanced diet, well-supplied with protein, carbohydrates, fats, and the necessary vitamins, there is no harm in including them in the diet. There is no longer a place for the time-worn theories that milk makes one sick; that pork is undesirable; that pie or cake is harmful; that all fat must be trimmed from meat and a only a small amount of butter used; that baseball player Enos Slaughter obtained his game-saving stamina from eating sunflower seeds and raisens; that Herb Elliott was able to run so well because he ate fruits and nuts; that fighter Tony Galento relied on beer

184

as a training diet; and that an athlete to become invincible must eat such concoctions as royal jelly ($40,000 worth a year), wheat-germ oil, black-strap molasses, and many other absurd foods. All such notions are plain nonsense. Physicians, coaches, and trainers could be doing their young athletes a lifelong service by combating such mistaken dietry practices. Fad feeding may have some magical value if it makes the athletes feel like heroes, but it is nonsense just the same.

THE PRE-GAME MEAL

One of the greatest problems for athletic coaches is not the pre-game meal, but rather the emotional make-up of the individual athlete who is to eat that meal. To offer a squad of 40 or 60 football players any given meal and expect all of their stomachs to react in the same way to the food is unreasonable. A coach can train a boy's will and muscles, but no one can dictate the emotional chemistry of his digestive juices. Many coaches believe in the theory that athletes should be a "little on the hungry" side before a contest. However, for physiological reasons some athletes can't keep their minds or bodies functioning properly without a solid meal (3 hours) before a ball game. Some athletes have superstitions of their own concerning food. For instance, youngsters whose parents come from certain sections of Europe still partake of the same pre-game meals they eat on nights they play at home. We all know of the Spanish-American children who have played well on a stomach full of chili. We also know that athletes of Scandinavian and German descent have a diet of rather heavy pastries. For nutritional efficiency these special environmental and personality requirements must be correlated with balanced diets. But to prohibit a boy from enjoying his home environment is to tamper with emotional desires that often are stronger than the influence of his Alma Mater. Former Olympic athletes tell about the peculiar diets they saw in the Olympic villages and of their surprise that the athletes were able to perform with great efficiency and without regurgitation.

The pre-game meal should possess an adequate total caloric load of 1,000 to 1,500 calories and should be well balanced with respect to carbohy-

185

drates, fats, and proteins. It must be eaten at least three hours before game time.

During the past few years other fads have received notice. One of these was Gatorade® which was developed by Shires and Bradley of the University of Florida and marketed by Stokely-Van-Camp. The known ingredients of this concoction include: citric acid, salt, glucose, water, .040 per cent sodium carboxymethylcellulose (non-nutritive), Sodium Orthophosphate, .053 per cent calcium cyclamate (non-nutritive), potassium chloride, gum acacia, potassium orthophosphate, sodium bicarbonate, natural and artificial flavor, artificial color, nd .005 per cent Sodium saccharin (non-nutritive). Many have sung the praise of Gatorade.® The University of Florida is said to have won nine football games in one recent season, and Gatorade® was credited as the principal reason. It has been claimed further that the two losses that Florida sustained during that same year were due to the unavailability of the concoction on those two occasions — once when a bulldog drank the barrelfull and another when a hurricane blew the barrel away.

It would seem from a medical standpoint that the salt and water content, which is important in avoiding heat stroke, and a little sweetener may actually be the components of the solution that cause the athletes to perform better. Doctor Fred Allman, Jr. reported that "one college in the Southeast, whose coach later became a General in the Army, had a large barrel of sauerkraut just out side the dressing room and all football players were encouraged to eat freely from the barrel each day." Allman further notes that a certain player would bring a case of Coca-Cola® to the courtside during a match and drink most of it during the course of the match.

CARBOHYDRATES

The major part of the caloric requirement for body growth and function is furnished by carbohydrates, with protein and fats playing a secondary role. Studies have shown that a high carbohydrate diet yields a 5 per cent greater muscular efficiency than a high protein or high fat diet. Carbohydrates are stored in the form of glycogen in the liver and muscles, where it represents a readily available source of energy. During prolonged physical activity a decrease in the glycogen stores is accompanied by an increase in the symptoms of fatigue. When sugar is fed, these symptoms disappear. Studies on marathon runners showed that following a race there was always a marked fall of blood sugar. It was observed that the state of the exhausted runner was similar to that in progressive insulin shock. It is for this reason that marathon runners take sweets in adequate amounts before and during the race. The athlete victim of hypoglycemia may have such symptoms as nervousness, mild headache, anxiety, tension, and irritability which may seriously affect his coordination and endurance. However, some athletes are hypersensitive to dietary sugars. Feeding them large amounts of sugars in the hope of providing quick energy or high efficiency may have an opposite effect to that desired. In individuals hypersensitive to dietary sugars a slight rise in blood sugar stimulates the pancreatic cells to overproduce insulin, causing a mild state of hypoglycemia. This may also happen to a normal individual who has an overdose of sugar, or may be the result of hunger when the pre-game meal was eaten too long before competition, or was insufficient in quantity. Such a mild state of hypoglycemia may take the athlete irritable and uncooperative.

The fat portion of the athlete's diet should **not** be more than double that of carbohydrate. If dietary carbohydrate is inadequate some of the fatty acids are not oxidized. A toxic acidosis may result which will lower the body defenses to fatigue.

OTHER DIETARY FACTORS

Dietary proteins are important for athletes since they furnish not only important organic constituents of muscles, but also of glandular tissues and blood plasma. In addition, they may also enhance the development of resistance to infections, the healing of wounds, and good functioning of the liver. Thus, the major role of proteins in the body is the construction and preservation of the integrity of body tissues.

Milk and milk products are the best source of calcium for athletes. Some calcium is also present in green vegetables and some fruits. Some fractures sustained by athletes have been due to weakened bones, caused by a lack of calcium in their diet.

Sweating is a nutritional problem because it robs the body of salt. A salt loss as low as 5 per cent will cause lassitude and fatigue, while a loss of between 40 and 50 per cent will cause heat cramps and prostration. Salt tablets should be given to athletes who sweat a great deal on hot days.

SUMMARY

The following eight points are important to the young athlete:

1. A well balanced selection of fruits, vegetables, meats, and dairy products will supply all the necessary fats, carbohydrates, proteins, and minerals needed for any conceivable activity. Any elaborate supplements are not necessary, and exotic side dishes add nothing useful to the diet.

2. Regular elimination of waste products is essential.

3. Adequate rest of both mind and body must be obtained.

4. A sense of humor is the best antidote for tension.

5. Excessive emotional tension which leads to personal ineffectiveness should be avoided.

6. The mutual loyalty of fellow players, friends, and family is desirable.

7. The athlete's pride in his position on the team is a great asset.

8. Continued growth in knowledge, wisdom, and experience lead to maturity.

REFERENCES

[1]Allman, F. L., Jr.: Quackery in Sports — Foolishness and Folklore. Personal Communication

[2]Trickett, P. S.: Athletic Injuries. World-Wide absts. 8:10, June 1965

[3]Guild, W. R.: How to Keep Fit and EnJoy It. Revised Edition. Simon and Schuster, Inc., New York, 1967

Weight Control in Athletics

HERMAN C. MAGANZINI, MD, FACP

It has been shown experimentally that obese individuals expend more energy for each unit of work performed, when compared to normal controls. There is also an increase in the "relative intensity" of energy expenditure for moderate work, ie, the blood pressure, heart rate, pulmonary ventilation, and alveolar-arteriolar PO_2 difference is increased in these individuals per unit of work.[1] In addition, it has been shown that obese individuals adapt poorly to heat and may not acclimatize at all under those same conditions of fluid and salt intake, plus exercise in the heat, which would produce this in those of normal weight.

In essence, the athlete best able to perform his given task in any sport, would be one of the proper weight and muscular development for his height and body build, given of course the necessary conditioning, coordination and skills.

Body Composition

When we speak of body weight we ordinarily give little consideration to what this represents in detail. The "scale weight" is really a composite of all those parts of the body which contribute to the body mass, namely fat, muscle, water, bone and other tissues. The weight of bone and other fixed tissue cannot readily be changed and, therefore, are not pertinent to the present discussion. The various proportions of fat, muscle, and water in an individual *can* be modified and are important to his functional capacity.

Body Water

In males 65% of the body weight is water. The specific percentage depends on the lean body mass, for adipose tissue (fat) contains only 20% water, while muscle contains 75% water. Obviously the more muscular individual would have a greater proportion of body water when compared to the fat one. Most of this water is inside of the body cells (intracellular) and under most considerations remains relatively stable at approximately 41% of the body weight. Of the other 24% (extra-cellular fluid), 4% is in the plasma (the liquid part of the blood), 15% is in the interstitial space (those minute crevices between cells and tissue planes), and 5% in the other areas (bone, water, eye fluid, etc.). Under ordinary circumstances water balance is maintained by the intake of approximately 1200 cc as the liquid part of food, 300 cc produced by the metabolism of this food to carbon dioxide and water, and 1000 cc in the form of actual liquid drinks. Of this ingested amount, approximately 1500 cc is excreted as urine, with 150 cc in the stool, while 350 cc is lost in the expired air, and 500 cc by "insensible perspiration". This is not actual *sweat* as we usually appreciate it but minute quantities lost constantly from the skin and not really felt by us. This is a total output balancing the intake of approximately 2500 cc. Most increases in intake are balanced by automatic physiologic mechanisms which increase the output of urine. Marked increases in water loss, such as visible sweat, can only be balanced by voluntary increases in the intake of fluid and salt.[2]

Fat (Adipose Tissue)

Calories ingested in excess of daily needs are stored as fat. Those calories greater than the energy expended in heat production or in work are so stored. The caloric value of human adipose tissue (fat) has been calculated at approximately 3500 calories per pound, ie, one pound of fat will yield 3500 calories when metabolized.[3] This means that

190

in order to lose one pound of fat, sufficient energy must be expended to utilize 3500 calories more than consumed as food or drink during the same time interval. Likewise, in order to gain one pound of fat an individual must consume food with a caloric value of 3500 calories greater than that used.

Muscle

Muscle is that tissue which actually performs the work of exercise and of productive work. All athletic training is aimed towards developing many or specific groups of muscle peculiar to the sport in question. This is in addition of course to the general cardiovascular adaptations of conditioning which are essential and common to well trained athletes in any sport.

Weight Change

Increase or decrease in weight can be reasonably accomplished only by manipulating the variables of water and fat *primarily,* and less so that of muscle mass. Loss of muscle weight occurs only in malnutrition or in the changes which occur when the highly developed muscular individual becomes less well developed and untrained as he stops continuous exercise or work. Even then the total body weight may not necessarily decrease but frequently remains stable as the ratio of fat to muscle changes. Some part of the weight which previously had been muscle is now fat. Well trained and muscular athletes especially in certain sports such as football and the shot-putter in track, etc. tend to have large well developed muscle masses. We are all aware however of the 225 pound, 6 foot 2 inch college lineman who grows to a 225 pound flabby, desk worker some years later. What happened to him? His height and weight are the same but now the muscle mass previously developed by constant exercise and work is gone. This muscle weight loss has been masked however by a weight gain of fat. His non-playing ideal weight as compared to his ideal weight while muscularly active is probably closer to 200 pounds or less.

Gaining weight by building muscle on the other hand requires continuous exercise and work to develop those muscles in question. This is accomplished by weight lifting, running, etc. but even then there is frequently little weight gain but rather a replacement of the lost weight of fat by increasing muscle mass.

The other two variables of total body weight namely water and fat, are much more easily manipulated.

Water

Except following dehydration or certain abnormal physiological states, one does not ordinarily gain weight by an excessive ingestion of fluids. The normal compensatory mechanisms quickly cause excretion of the excessive amounts of fluid to restore equilibrium.

Inadequate intake of fluid however, especially if coupled with excessive loss of both water and salt (as can occur in August, September, and later in Maryland) can result in substantial weight loss. This is not however the type of weight loss which is beneficial to the player or coach and can certainly be detrimental and even dangerous to the point of death. Dehydration, that is the excessive loss of body water, can cause (in addition to weight loss) a decrease in plasma water with a decrease in blood volume followed by decreasing flow to the body tissues and therefore a decreased delivery of oxygen. In addition there is a decrease in the blood flow through the kidneys with decreased ability to excrete acids. Both of the latter cause an increase of acid accumulation within the body or the condition *acidosis*. The body temperature and heart rate rise, the output of the heart (cardiac output) falls and there is exhaustion and collapse.

In a hot and humid environment the loss of salt and water can cause heat cramps, heat exhaustion and finally if persistent and severe, heat stroke and death. The measuring of weight loss on a daily basis can be a valuable clue to the coach or trainer, especially in the early practices and games of the late summer and fall. Rapid fluctuations of more than one to two pounds are always due to changes in fluid balance. All candidates should be weighed before and after each practice session. Any boy losing more than five pounds, which amounts to approximately ten quarts of body fluid, must be carefully watched. Any individual approaching a ten pound weight loss (20 qt of fluid) must be especially watched, controlled, instructed and very severely restricted if necessary. This is an individual bordering on the dangerous fluid losses preceding heat stroke. Free access to water or preferably dilute salt solution on the field during all practices and games must be assured, and a priming dose should be encouraged during the suiting up period. Salt tablets and salt solutions should be encouraged and provided. The other precautions of temperature, humidity and uniform previously outlined should be followed.[4]

The changes in weight due to water loss are primarily important in order to avoid dehydration, heat exhaustion and possibly heat stroke.

Fat

Here, really, is the weight controlling variable of which we are all really thinking when this subject is being considered. The previous points were made primarily to keep one reminded that putting a boy on the scale does not necessarily measure only fat tissue loss or gain but also the other variables. As mentioned previously, this fat tissue is deposited whenever caloric intake exceeds utilization. Energy is needed by the body first for what is called *basal metabolism*. These are the basic needs of life namely to maintain body temperature, to maintain the autonomic (automatic) functions of the body such as the heartbeat, respirations, gut function, etc. and then the synthetic tissue reaction such as forming proteins and the other chemical reactions of the body. One requires energy also to perform the daily activities which are not really productive work but still essential, such as feeding and clothing. The last portion of energy expenditure is that which is essential in performing one's daily work whatever it may be.

The basic metabolic functions consume about 1500 calories daily (500 while asleep and 1000 while awake) while the daily necessary activities require approximately another 500. These 2000 calories are needed to perform *non-labor activities. Work activities* may vary from 600 calories for a really sedentary individual to as high as 3000 calories (approximately) for a really active athlete.

The caloric value of food consumed varies with its composition. Carbohydrate develops four calories per gram as does protein whereas each gram of fat consumed produces more than twice as much—nine calories per gram. Ethanol (alcohol) delivers approximately seven calories per gram. It is extremely easy with the usual adolescent diet to exceed the 2500 calorie requirement for sedentary and even the 3500 to 4000 calories of the athlete. It only takes a few milkshakes, french fries, hamburgers, chocolate bars plus the usual feedings to accomplish this and therefore gain weight. It is obviously more difficult to lose one pound of *fat weight* which requires the utilization of 3500 calories in excess of intake. This implies that the decreased intake of calories is essential in any program of true fat tissue loss almost in spite of the exercise program involved.

Adjuncts

Diet Pills: Although these may be helpful in decreasing appetite under ordinary circumstances they are contraindicated in the actively training individual, especially during the heat acclimatization period of the fall. The secondary cardiovascular side effects and the reported deaths while taking these stimulant drugs in hot and humid weather make it essential that they not be used.

Special Foods: In spite of the obvious food faddism especially among some of our professional athletes there is, at the present time, no demonstrable, experimental proof that honey, wheat germ, rose hips, kelp, corn oil, etc. are helpful in increasing performance or stamina. I have never felt it essential however to insist that the athletes discontinue the use of these especially if the individual is convinced of their value. Conversely, coaches, trainers, and physicians should not encourage these supplements since they certainly are not helpful and perhaps place wrong emphasis on their value versus training. Some of these foods in addition, cause gastrointestinal upset and it would seem foolish to risk nausea, vomiting or indigestion prior to an athletic contest in order to gain a minimal psychologic and a nonexistent physiologic effect.

Vitamins: No vitamins have been shown helpful including injections of Vitamin B-12, high potency B vitamins, Vitamin E, etc., etc., etc. in spite of what is written in the lay press and in spite of what some trainers and even the physicians of some teams seem to encourage.

Salt: It is essential to have salt supplied in large quantities along with adequate fluid in the training and acclimatization periods. Once again this is not one of the things that can be done on the day of a game. The salt and fluid stores of the body have to be built up over the ten days to two weeks which are necessary for heat acclimatization in order to be valuable. It is not worth risking nausea and vomiting in pushing salt pills on an individual the day of the game. The athlete must be encouraged to take the salt as tablets and in liberal quantities on food during the training period. Much more essential is the provision of adequate fluid in liberal and unrestricted quantities on the field for the game, perhaps in the form of palatable salt solution but even as water.

Pre-game Meals: Depending on the state of excitement and the type of food (such as fat versus carbohydrate versus protein) it will take two to six hours or longer for the stomach to empty following a meal. The only advantage of a liquid meal might be if it were more easily digested and tolerated, without nausea or vomiting. Regardless of the long history of traditional meals prior to a game that many teams use, physiologically nothing ingested on the morning of the game (or between halves of the football game) will have any effect on performance. A proper diet during the previous days and weeks building up glycogen stores, etc. is much more important to adequate performance on the day of the game.

Ideal Weight: The ideal weight for any individual varies depending on height, body stature and muscular development. It varies somewhat from sport to sport. Comparing a long distance runner with a football interior lineman as to adequate and ideal weight, using the same standards, would obviously be unreasonable for their muscular development is entirely different. We are considering muscle weight and not a *flabby fat boy.* There are many tables available, some of them quite elaborate including hip measurements, chest measurements, etc. but simple height and weight tables usually suffice. Most often a coach or trainer can look at one of his candidates and tell whether or not it is fat or muscle in the overweight suspect. There is a tendency among some football coaches to like *'heft* in their line regardless of whether it is fat or muscle. I think however, most of the better coaches would agree that usually a 210 pound fat boy is going to be moved by a 190 pound muscular, agile individual of the same size.

As far as wrestlers and their coaches are concerned, we have another problem. They are interested primarily in what the lowest weight would be to allow the athlete to compete in the lightest category possible. This varies of course with stature but the various devices used in the past and even the present to make the "weigh in" are to be deplored. As is obvious from our previous discussion rapid weight losses are always due to water and salt loss. These deficits of dehydration cannot be repaired within the several hours prior to a match and still expect the athlete to perform well or even safely. Nor is it reasonable to keep a boy on a semi-starvation or dehydrating diet to help him stay within a given weight class and expect him to perform safely.

Can anything be done to avoid the weigh-in problems especially of a sport such as wrestling? Should weighing in before matches be completely abolished? A recommendation has been made that all boys out for wrestling be weighed on a surprise weigh-in twice a year, placed in a weight category and left there for the rest of the year regardless of change. Another plan would weigh the wrestler after four to six weeks of training and make that his minimum effective weight.[5] Some change may be due!

Summary

Obesity is undesirable in any athlete for it impairs his ability to perform to the maximum of his own personal, ultimate capabilities.

True (fat) weight loss can only be attained by hard physical work and decreased food intake, especially of the high caloric foods, so that the energy expended is in excess of the calories ingested at the rate of 3500 calories per pound of fat.

Special foods, such as honey, wheat germ, etc. are of no help and should not be encouraged. For an individual who is already convinced of their efficacy and using them, controversy can be avoided unless they are shown to cause him gastrointestinal upset or other detriment.

No diet pills, Vitamin B-12, anabolic steroids, etc. are necessary or desirable. Certain of these can cause toxicity and be detrimental.

No rubber suits should be encouraged or tolerated for they do not cause true fat weight loss but only fluid loss and have been implicated in precipitating heat stroke.

Rapid weight fluctuations of any magnitude are due to fluid shifts and do not represent *fat* weight loss or gain and therefore are not of themselves desirable. Chronic or acute dehydration can be extremely dangerous to the athlete, especially so in hot, humid weather.

I hope that all of the coaches, trainers, physicians and educators present will give serious consideration to the problems of weight in our athletes. Although obesity is undesirable, the opposite viz. artificially induced and excessive weight loss by dehydration and semistarvation is to be condemned. We must all be alert to safeguarding the individual above all, even to the detriment of the team if necessary. Standards must be reviewed, modified or discarded if unsuitable. These standards must be so arranged that all teams can compete without unfair advantage, and without compromising the safety of the individual athlete.

REFERENCES

1. Dempsey, J. A., Reddan, W., Balke, B. and Rankin, J.: Work Capacity Determinants and Physiologic Cost of Weight-Supported Work in Obesity." *J of Appl Physiol* **21**:1815-20, November 1966.

2. Murphy, R. J. and Asle, W. F.: "Prevention of Heat Illness in Football Players." *JAMA* **194**:650-654, 8 Nov 1965.

3. Best, C. H. and Taylor, N. B.: *The Physiologic Basis of Medical Practice.* Eighth Edition. Baltimore: Williams and Wilkins Co., 1966.

4. Maganzini, H. C.: "Heat Adaptation and Injury in Football Players." *Md Med J* **16**:45-49, October 1967.

5. "Wrestling and Weight Control." AMA Committee on Medical Aspects of Sports. *JAMA* **201**:541-543, 14 August 1967.

AUTHOR INDEX

KEY-WORD TITLE INDEX